M

An Alabama Midwife's Story

By Onnie Lee Logan as told to Katherine Clark

Untreed
Reads

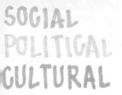

SOCIAL
POLITICAL
CULTURAL

Motherwit: An Alabama Midwife's Story

By Onnie Lee Logan as told to Katherine Clark

Copyright 2014 by Katherine Clark

Cover Design by Ginny Glass

ISBN-13: 978-1-61187-926-1

Published by Untreed Reads, LLC

506 Kansas Street, San Francisco, CA 94107

http://www.untreedreads.com

Previously published in print, 1989 and 1991

Previously published in ebook, Untreed Reads, 2013

Printed in the United States of America

Publisher's Note

The publisher does not have any control over and does not assume any responsibility for author or third-party Web sites or their content.

"Onnie's riveting story touches the heartstrings.... My only criticism of this book is that it cannot go on and on. I loved it."

—James Mellon, editor, *Bullwhip Days: The Slaves Remember*

"A life well lived unfolds in this exuberant, unlettered telling of a midwife's story.... In Logan's rich, regional speech as she talks with Clark, a strong, faith-filled woman is heard; her eloquent memoir is vivid Americana."

—*Publishers Weekly*

"What makes this story special is its voice. *Motherwit* is an oral accounting told in the warm and compelling language of the rural South. It is not difficult to imagine sitting at the kitchen table while Ms. Logan peeled peaches for a cobbler and spoke just above a whisper about shotgun houses...'luminum washtubs...and pumpin' water outside."

—*New York Times Book Review*

"It's rare to find someone who loved her work as much as Mrs. Logan. For her, childbirth is life's greatest miracle. 'Ain't God beautiful? Makes me want to scream on how it all works.' *Motherwit* is the beautiful offspring of her dedication to that miracle."

—*Atlanta Jounal Constitution*

"A rich story of black southern rural life."

—*Boston Herald*

* * *

ONNIE LEE LOGAN practiced midwifery in Alabama from 1931 to 1984. She was the last lay midwife practicing in Mobile. She told her story to Katherine Clark, an English professor at the University of Alabama in Tuscaloosa.

Contents

*Therefore God dealt well
with the midwives: and the
people multiplied, and
waxed very mighty.*
—Exodus 1:20

Introduction

The work that follows is the text of an oral autobiography told to me by a black granny midwife in Mobile, Alabama, during August 1984. Many white Mobilians knew Onnie Lee Logan only as a maid who for many years was an integral part of a prominent family's household, and it was through these people that I came to know her. Onnie always regarded midwifery as her real life's work, however, and the inspiration for this project came not from me, but from her overwhelming desire "not to die with it," as she said—not to die without sharing the "wisdom and knowledge" but especially the stories from her lifetime of experience. Onnie, a semiliterate woman with little formal education, told me she was "gonna write this book" if she "had to scratch it out" herself. "I got so much experience in here that I just want to explode," she told me. "I want to show that I knew what I knew—I want somebody to realize what I am." Hers is the story not only of midwifery, but of her personal odyssey as a rural black woman determined to lead a life of meaning and fulfillment.

Onnie Lee Logan was born around 1910, the fourteenth of sixteen children in Sweet Water, Marengo County, Alabama. Like all her brothers and sisters before her, Onnie was delivered by a midwife. Indeed, in that year, one-half of all births in America were attended by unlicensed, untrained midwives. In Alabama, Onnie's mother was one of these midwives. Onnie's grandmother, who had been a slave on a nearby plantation, had also been a midwife. Inspired by the stories about her

i

grandmother, by the example of her mother, and by the gospel of service her family instilled in her, Onnie decided as a young girl to become a midwife herself.

Lay midwives like Onnie's mother and grandmother, known by the community as "grannies," were simply women experienced in assisting other women during labor and childbirth. Midwifery began centuries ago and persevered through time as little more than the practice of childbearing women calling upon other women in their community to serve as birth attendants. Even in twentieth-century America, midwifery had not departed from its age-old origins. At the time when midwives were delivering one-half of all babies born in the United States, there were no training programs to educate midwives and no laws in any state to regulate their practice. Childbirth and midwifery both took place outside the realms of law and medicine.

Soon after 1910, when the United States discovered it had the third-highest infant and maternal mortality rates in the world, midwifery came under heavy attack. Doctors called for the elimination of midwives and the growth of obstetrics as the only way to impose standards for the care of pregnant women and newborns. They agreed the midwife should have no place in modern medicine, but also conceded that midwifery was a necessary evil until the practice of obstetrics became universal. While promoting the gradual abolition of all midwifery, they proposed for the interim a plan of midwife control and education.

By 1930, this plan was so well under way that only 15 percent of all births in America were attended by midwives, who were now regulated by laws and trained by boards of health in most states. Significantly, 80 percent of these midwives lived in the South, where physicians had always been extremely scarce and the population had the highest percentage of black, poor, and rural citizens. In 1915, for example, the progressive state of Massachusetts had been able to outlaw midwifery altogether. On the other hand, in 1919, Alabama was just passing its first law to *regulate* midwifery. Because of its unique cultural circumstances, the South was decades behind the rest of the country in establishing obstetrics for the care of all childbearing women. Midwifery became a Southern black phenomenon, and the South became the repository of the so-called midwife problem in America.

Each Southern state varied in its treatment of this "problem." Alabama's 1919 law officially recognized midwifery and placed it under control of the county boards of health. At first, many counties did little more than register midwives. Gradually, a more complete system developed in the bureaus of child hygiene and public health nursing. Potential midwives received instruction from public health nurses; were given written examinations; were subjected to monthly inspections of their equipment bags, their person, and their homes; were required to attend monthly meetings; and were expected to comply with all the stipulations concerning equipment, uniform, and personal hygiene. In addition, they could attend only normal deliveries. Ten years after the passage of the law, the essentials of this system were intact in most counties in Alabama.

Nevertheless, doctors and health officials in Alabama as in other Southern states would never be happy with any midwife program. It was the Southern states, with their high rates for blacks, that were largely responsible for making the national infant- and maternal-mortality rates so high. The medical establishment in the South condemned the "ignorant" black granny midwife as the source of the problem and began to work diligently toward establishing universal obstetrical care for indigent and rural blacks and whites.

In 1947, when Onnie wanted to become a midwife in Mobile County, Alabama had the highest maternal mortality rate in the nation. Midwives were attending one-fifth of all births and one-half of all black births in Alabama annually. To receive her license, Onnie had to undergo a nine-month training program and then submit to rigorous supervision and regulations from the board of health for annual renewal of her permit. For instance, her patients were required by law to receive prenatal care from a doctor, who then signed a release for home delivery, but was expected to come to Onnie's aid if she ran into difficulties or emergencies.

During her first eighteen years as a midwife, Onnie's patients were mostly poor black mothers living in Prichard and Crichton, the black areas of Mobile. She also attended many poor white mothers who lived in the rural areas of Mobile County. This type of clientele was traditional for the black granny midwife.

By the mid-1960s, the number of maternity clinics had finally caught up with the needs of rural and indigent patients, and Alabama's maternal and infant mortality rates had decreased dramatically. When the Maternal and Infant Care (MIC) clinic was established in Mobile, the number of Onnie's patients also decreased dramatically. After this time, those who engaged Onnie's services were usually lower-middle-class white fundamentalists who wanted their babies delivered in the same way that Moses had been—by a midwife.

Those white patients who could afford a hospital delivery began having difficulties getting their doctors to sign the release for home birth. Some doctors openly complained about being deprived of a delivery fee. At the same time, many physicians' partnerships were beginning to institute policies against signing releases for midwife delivery because of the malpractice liability involved.

In 1976, granny midwifery was outlawed in Alabama. Onnie was allowed to continue practicing until 1984, when she received a rather abrupt letter from the board of health indicating that there was no longer a "need" for her services and that her permit would not be renewed. She was the last granny midwife in Mobile and one of the last in Alabama.

Despite an impeccable record as a granny midwife, Onnie was stripped of her vocation and barred from performing a service as old as the human race. She had prepared herself to serve a need that existed in the rural, black, impoverished Alabama where she was born. But while she was becoming a midwife, the world that had called her into service was changing into one that did not want or "need" her. In 1931, a doctor in Magnolia, Alabama, had told her she would make a good midwife. Fifty years later, a doctor in Mobile told her it was a shame that she never became a physician. Caught in the flux of a changing culture, Onnie made for a very unusual victim of historical "progress." She faithfully and successfully served one world only to be told by the next that she was no longer needed.

Ironically, in 1989, Alabama's maternal and infant mortality rates are now again among the highest in the nation. The severe shortage of obstetricians appears to be responsible for the problem. In Alabama, as in many other parts of the country, doctors are leaving obstetrics in droves because of malpractice liability. In many rural Alabama counties today, there are no obstetrical services available whatsoever. Sometimes women in labor must drive for hours to reach the nearest hospital that provides obstetrical care. One solution currently under serious consideration is the establishment of a nurse midwife program. And so the history of midwifery may have come full circle.

Onnie's story is a part of this history. But more important, this is the story of the personal triumph of a Southern black woman so proud of what she had done with her life that she felt compelled to share it with the world.

—Katherine Clark

Beginnings

My name is Onnie Lee Logan. I was born in Sweet Water Alabama in Marengo County. To tell you the truth, I don't exactly know what age I am. I have never had a birth certificate. In those days—I think it was somewhere about 1910—they didn't really keep an accurate record for black people. I don't know why not. To my point, I would think they never paid us too much attention anyway other than getting the work out of us. As far as a record and all that concerned, I just don't think it was there. They ain't got a certificate on me. I feel like this year my birthday I was seventy-three. Now it could be more or less. It could be more or less. That's true.

In Sweet Water there was a Mr. Jack Maynard. He was a white man, called my mother Tinny. That was Mother's nickname. My mother did washin for him. She was carryin me and he said, "Tinny, you let me name that baby if it's a girl and I'll buy it some dresses." When Mother told him all right he named me after his wife who had passed. Her name was Onnie.

My father's father was Indian. My daddy was not a black Negro. He was not. He was an Indian at least two-thirds of the way. My father looked more like a Indian than any black man you ever seen. You'd said he was full-blooded Indian. He was a big, stout, nice-lookin, light-skinned Indian man. Beautiful hair. Beautiful straight hair. Not completely straight, but all you had to do was brush it real good. You can put a lil oil in it, just a lil oil, and then brush it so pretty. You know I used to cut his hair all the time. His sister, my aunt Mandy, she wore her hair parted in the middle and platted in two plats. That's the only way she could wear it is to plain braid it in two big tails. She had those great big tits and the pigtails hangin down right over em.

All of us had the soft hair. Usually it sheds. You know the Indians how it sheds out thin the older they get. Sheds thin. That's the reason my hair the older I get the thinner my hair get. If I'm goin to church and I want to wear a hat I have to put a wig on it now cause I cain't wear a hat with no more hair than I got. My granddaddy and my grandmother they was both light-complexioned Indians. It wasn't the dark kind. We got most of our darkness on our mother's side which she had Indian in her too. But there was different Indians. Creek and Choctaw. So my daddy was one and my mother was the other. My mother her part Indian she was the dark. That's the Creek Indians.

I never did see my father's father. He was married to a midwife. All I got was from my daddy and my mother and my old aunt, Aunt Mandy. They told me my grandfather was an Indian. I got that when I's quite a lil girl. The words you know. What they be talkin about. These are the same ones that talked about my grandmother the midwife. She was also part Indian and she was a slave. I don't know if my grandfather was a slave. I think that in that time everybody that wasn't white was a slave. Even the Indians. You know how they did em.

My grandfather gave to Daddy before my time land. He give him a start at life. He put a deed in my father's name. I have no way in the world to know how my grandfather got that land. All I know is he had it. I don't know whether his old slave daddy give it to him or how he come about it. I don't know nothin in this world about my grandfather. I just know what was told to me about him. That he gave Dad his start. And what a fine man he was. Cause we had land. Long befo I was, he gave him property. When I knew my daddy he had the land. It was there. I was told from a child that my granddaddy whom I don't know give that. When I came into know, we had as much land as we could work plus there was cow pasture. Two big pastures. One for the mules and one for the cows. We didn't have to work that. Grazin land. My daddy just kep it a'goin. He always added to it. And worked that lil land he had.

I know we had mo than the other black families in Sweet Water. Our parents didn't tell us nothin. They raised us right. But I know. A lot a people had whatcha call sharecroppin. They didn't have land. In sharecroppin you workin the other fellow's land. I work for you and half I make you get and I get the other lil half. Or you get two-thirds and I get a third. They worked the other men's property for to make a livin and then that's when what they made had to be sharecropped to pay that man. We didn't have that. My grandmother, they had that to do after the Civil War. Sometime they would make just about enough to carry them through the winter. That's about three months or fo until it's time to start back again. We really didn't have that to do. I don't remember sharing crop any. I ain't never heard my daddy say he sharecropped. The others it was not their own property. "John, you almost got outa debt this time." I done heard that so much and I know that so much until it just was. "You almost made it." Then left em with nothin but probably about enough corn to make meal, make bread and some of those sour molasses and maybe a lil cane. Some potatoes and peas. Dried peas to eat off all winter. I'm not kiddin you. And a lot of em didn't have that. No I'm not kiddin you one bit. The black had done paid off long ago. A lot a times the reason they did that was to keep em from movin off. Movin on to somebody's else's place. "You still owe me. You got to stay and work with me next year. Cause you still owe me." That's exactly the way it was. Everybody. I could hear. In those days, Mother and them didn't let us in on everything. They didn't tell their impo'tant business of the adults. But we could hear it. "Mr. So-and-So and them they didn't make enough cotton to pay himself out this year. They didn't do this. They still owe the man so much and so much and so much." Heard that.

They had some animals. They raised their chickens, their hogs. Plenty of em didn't have as much food as us. Mother didn't give em time to come. She would take em vegetables, she would take em meal, flour, piece of meat, whatever. They acted fine because what we had—if my daddy killed a hog or a cow or somethin like that for meat, we always had enough to share. Love, care, and share, that's what we did. We had it and my daddy and mother they shared with the ones that didn't have it. Mother would send a piece and share.

My father, we had this huge plantation and we farmed. Durin my time comin up a lil girl when I first knew my family, they always was about three mules and two horses in the family to work with. There was always from eight to ten cows to be milked all the time. There was always a yoke of ox. My brother

4

Curtis, one a my oldest brothers, he just loved that. He died almost foolin with them ox to haul logs with those old red big wheels. He did that. My daddy raised them oxes. Those cows were raised from our milk cows. I cain't never remember when we didn't have from fo on up cows to milk. We had goats, cows, turkeys, guineas, ducks, hogs, horses, mules—they were there. We made our livin all off the farm because we had everything as far as eatable from cows, sheeps, hogs, and goats. Chickens— you couldn't walk in the yard. My mother, we would raise chickens and little bittys. We had a chicken yard fenced in so they couldn't get out cause there was so many of em. I declare I'd walk through there and step on little bittys and kill them a many day. There was so many of em you didn't have nowhere to step. Didn't mean to do it but it was so many of em. Bout three and fo hundred in the chicken yard at times, especially in the spring when they hatch out.

My mother in those days know how to pickle beef and meat and keep it. If she wanted to keep some fresh she would put it in a big lard can and shut it up and let it down in that deep well to the water. It's so fur down in the ground it could keep two or three days. We had a smokehouse with hams and millions of everything. Hams by ham. Those bacon millions we had all of that from one end in here to the other where they smoked. Sausage—we made our own sausage. We smoke em just like smoke sausage you buy at the sto. We had that year-round. We would go in there and slice ham and have for breakfast and a slice of bacon. We'd go in there and slice off for to boil the vegetables.

We had so many of us we had three big gardens. String beans, butter beans, turnip greens, English peas, sweet potatoes, Irish potatoes, okra, ever'thing. Tomatoes, three or fo different kinds of squash. Everything that was plantable we planted. I'd be havin to name every kind of vegetable there was to name what all we had. We had a peach o'chard. Peaches, pears, plums, preserves, and jelly. We made our own syrup. Syrup would last for a month way over the time we had to make syrup for another year. My daddy dug out a place about fo feet in the ground and then built a lil house up over it. About fo feet down and made shelves around in there. You know why he dug it like that? To keep it from freezin in the wintertime. You see that heat come up. That's the way we did. All the way around down in the ground on the ground part was three and fo and five hundred jars of fruit and vegetables. That's the way it was.

I've known when we've had two cribs as big as this and from here up down, we had that much co'n together every year. Mostly two cribs full. We had meal co'n. We make our own grits. Take it to the mill. Dependin on how they set the rock you could get different things from the co'n. You can get meal. You can get grits and you can get cracked co'n. The cracked co'n was just barely cracked—chicken feed. If I had a grain of co'n now and I cracked it and it come a'loose into two or three lil parts, that's cracked co'n. So we eat that. Kep the meal and the co'n cracked up like grits. And up in the loft—had a loft—we fill that full of hay for the ho'ses and the cows and the mules.

We grew rice, our own rice. There's a great big swamp down there and all we had to do was to get in there with our mules and them oxes and turn em over and get a handful of rice down like that. Just a handful. You didn't have to work that. It just come up in big bunches. When it got ripe we'd go in there and tie them big bunches together and cut em off and carry em and put em in that big long hole. Level flo. When it get dry we would hit it up against the wall and make it shell out. Make the rice fall off from the stalk part of it.

We had this great big thing that Daddy would put gallons of em at a time in that thing and beat it. A rice beater we always called it. He cut an oak tree down and got a big stump off of it and sit that stump up. Then he hewed out as much as he could with his chisel in the center of it. Tryin to make a hole in the middle of that stump. After he couldn't chisel as much as he could to make it even then he set a fire in there and burned it as fur as he wanted to. He chiseled out almost as deep as he wanted and then he burned it. After burnin he sand it out and made it smooth, good and smooth.

Then he made what we call a maul. It was a round piece of wood with a stick on it. He would take that around and put the rice in there in the stump. Put the rice in there in the stump and then we would take that maul and beat it up and down on the top of the rice. They'd let it fall in the pan down into another pan. Every once in a while we'd put our hands through it to see if all the husks, all the rice had gotten outa the husks. That's a windy day. A windy day is when we beat enough rice could last you—you know how you could keep rice—forever. So a big windy day then we'd take that rice and spread a sheet out and then take it in a bucket and hold it up high. Let the rice fall down on the sheet and the husks would blow off. The wind would blow. We did that mo than one time to get all the husks and the rice was just as pretty and white as the rice that you buy at the sto. Mother would keep it in a can so we could use rice. Have rice when we got ready. It had to be a windy day cause the wind had to blow that husks. If it wasn't a windy day, Lord he'p us because we was so smart. Jesus, God knows it. The ones would get a big pastebo'd and fan it. They blow it cause the husks was nothing but lil light husks. It would easy blow off if we needed rice and didn't have a windy day. That's the way we lived. Not very many people grew rice cause you would have to go get the seed and plant it.

My father loved to come to Mobile and he would come to Mobile. Barges from Nanafalia to Mobile. It would come all the way from Demopolis down to Nanafalia then all the way down Tombigbee on in to Mobile. When I remembered him he was makin trips every so often to Mobile. Use to all I could hear him talkin about when I's a lil girl—Mardi Gras. Now that's when he come to Mobile. He loved that. Him and certain lot a friends they would all come to Mobile. He would come back with everything he could get his hands on. That's where he got our rice.

Two or three lil bales of cotton—that didn't include us. We made about twelve and fifteen and fo'teen. We made cotton. A lot of it. Indeed. Co'se in those times it wasn't sellin for a whole lot now. But we made whatever it cost. Whatever it was paid for we made it. We couldn't borrows off three or fo bales of cotton in a run of a year. Ain't never known us to make that lil. My daddy didn't have anybody else to help him with all them chil'ren. Sixteen of us and we got grown up like that. He had all the help he needed. We had to do everything that come to hand on the farm. I had hard-workin parents and they raised us as hard-workin chil'ren.

When I was young, comin up eight, nine, and ten until I's a young girl, I was the sickly one and I couldn't stay in the hot sun so I didn't work in the field like the rest of em. I couldn't stand that hot sun. I fainted a lot. I'd just fall off. I never will fo'get the day they carried me one day in the buggy, or was it a surrey? We had a buggy, surrey, and wagon. Mother carried me to the doctor because I kep fallin off and faintin. He told her then I'd always do this off and on but when I get to be a young lady I'd get rid of all that. I would stay home and cook and I would make these dresses for em to go to work in. I would sew old muslin gingham dresses. That was all there was in those days. I would sew in the mornin's, most of the mornin's, and then in the afternoon I have the dinner done for all of em.

My mother would go around and supervise em cause she had her babies so fast there wasn't much she could do and my father didn't want her out there workin. I don't know exactly but I believe she was about fifteen when she got married. The main meal was lunch, or as we called it dinner. We would have for breakfast we would have either hot biscuits and ham or bacon or syrup or rice or grits. Then for dinner we had three or fo different kinds of vegetables with the pure meat cooked in it.

9

Sometime if Mother was go'n stay home and help do it we would kill two or three chickens and make chicken and dumplin's. At suppertime I'll tell you the truth. This was really the routine. Most our suppers we'd have co'nbread and milk. A light supper. And sometimes we would have vegetables left over from dinner in the middle of the day. The ones that wanted that would have that.

On our plantation it wasn't much money. Wasn't a whole lot. Daddy made no progress on a whole lot a money but he kep it goin. We were makin a livin. It didn't take a whole lot a money to live in those times. Long about that time there wasn't no great wealthy white people either. They had money. They had somethin. Naturally. But I don't know of anybody livin in Sweet Water, back up in that area, that I would say was real wealthy. They had farms. They had mo but not a lot. You would say a New Yo'ker and people in these big cities was wealthy wealthy. But not in the country and Marengo County and Alabama. I know they lived well. I know they had this and they had that. But they had farms just like we did. They wasn't rollin over in money. Against somebody from New Yo'k, one these great big cities, they was mo on a level with us than they like to live with in their hearts and minds. That's where a lot of yo trouble be come in. There just wasn't a whole lot a money to be had long in those days. Either you had five dollars or you had five hundred. I'm not kiddin. But with them boys and them girls that grew up, didn't look like it take em very long to grow up. They kep some money comin in.

There were several white people that lived in different areas around our property, when we got through with our hoein and layin by our crop, we went to help them for money. We were hired out. We worked and were glad to work. Kep on our feet. Dad hired out the girls as well. I went. We'd hoe in the field or pick cotton in the field. We worked and were glad to work. Didn't know nothin else but work. When it come time to make a lil money I always tried to go then so I could make some money cause we spent our own money on ourselves. Buyin material to make us some clothes. Our socks that we wore to Sunday school. We helped our daddy with whatever it is to make it. You see we worked. That why I work now. That's why I always work now. Pickin cotton is back-breakin work but anybody used to it and know how it is and that's what they been doin can do it. You get tired but you go home and you go to bed and go to rest and you able to go again in the mornin. I have picked a hundred and fifty or a hundred and seventy-five pounds a day. But now I had a sister she would pull two hundred pounds all the time. We wouldn't make much cause there wasn't no money. It was just like everything else. Just like everything else. Along about that time they were payin about a dollar or seventy-five cents a day all day to pick that much cotton. Thirty-five cents, fo'ty cents. Then it went up fifty cents, a hundred. My brothers they would be hired out sometimes to help plow. Dad let us did it. He told us, "Mr. So-and-So want you all to come over there and hoe. You done finished yo cho'es and you can go over there to do that." Now and then if he caught up with his cottonin and didn't have nothin to do he would he'p plow. He would do that.

A lot a people in those days they made preserves outa blackberries. When we got through with the cotton and crop we'd pick those blackberries out our great big swamp down there and take em down to that sawmill quarter and sold em to those white people so they could make preserves. We would take that money and go buy material to make us a Sunday school dress.

My father would sell timber off his land. The boys would get out there and make cotton and all this co'n and when they laid by between crops they take the mules and get back out in them woods. By the cord they would cord that wood up. Down at the mill they showed them boys how to cord it up. They ran off the pine knots. There's a great big old steam train would go through Sweet Water and it run by pine knots. Daddy would get that cordwood to make money with. The boys would haul those pine knots to make their cash money and when there wasn't no money, ride on those old trains that went through there. Daddy had to buy the tractors and all the clothes and have to pay the fee to send us to school. Now if he thought he would run outa money he would go to the bank and borrow a lil money and go pay back at the end of the year when he sell his cotton. So after as many of us as it was we made a livin out of it and then Dad was able to save a lil. As my daddy grew and times got better and better he would buy mo land joinin that so he had a great big plantation. It was huge when he died.

Besides all a that, my father was a carpenter. You know, people in that area, far and near, white and black, my daddy made their caskets. He made em. You know, the casket used to be made sharp on the end out and then come sharp on this end. He made those caskets with his saw and hammer and got white material, or black material, and dressed em. Instead of havin the rough box they were colored and that material was tacked. He would take em over to the house himself in his wagon.

There was a sawmill quarter. Cox-Heap Sawmill. All that I know from my eyes there was lumber stacked up everywhere out there. Mr. Miller and Mr. Cox that owned that sawmill kep my daddy busy building lil houses for people to live in. White was on this side of the sawmill, and the colored people was on the other side. All those lil houses that they was livin in. They were just made outa rough lumber, plain lumber from the sawmill. Two to three rooms and fo sometimes. That was durin rough times. Two bedrooms and a kitchen. No livin rooms and no bathrooms. Each one had its own lil outhouse. When Daddy had the buildin to do, he did it and the chil'ren kep the crop goin cause that was cash money, such as it was. My daddy did not build our house. But now he built Amos a house. He built my sister Nettie a house. He built Elmer a house. Those houses he built for my brothers and sisters were on our property. He would do that for all of em when they got grown and married.

My mother would let those boys, me and a couple of my sisters get the mule and wagon and go and bring back from ten to twelve loads of clothes from that quarter to our house and wash em. We did washin for white people. Black people did their own. Some folded and ironed em and carried em back. Outa all them clothes, those clothes didn't get mixed up. You got part of my clothes and I got part of yo's. None a that.

13

Washed em, hung em up on a line and dried em, taken em off and ironed em, and carried em back home. Washin in tubs. In that time they had a few tin tubs but mostly they had these great big barrels, that you would saw in two and my daddy would put hooks around em and we kep water in em all the time so they swelled and the water never got dry or leaked out of em. You know if they dried they would crack where they were joined together. So we kep water in em all the time. And two big pots. They would wash them clothes first and then put em in these two big pots and boil em like ster'lizin em. Mostly in those days was Octagon soap that they used all the time. Real old time. My mother would make soap. Lye soap. She used that as well. The people that gave the clothes to us would send the soap and the starch cause people starched clothes in those days. Rinse em three times in the water and then hang em up on the line. Our clothesline was huge. About three or fo strings. Long, honey. From here all the way to I don't know where.

We had the irons that you sit up to the fire. The lil old-timey smoothin irons they call em. We knew exactly how hot to let it get and know how to iron it to keep from sco'chin it. I had a sister she was an old maid. Sweet old maid. She didn't get married until she was in her late fifties. That girl could iron, I'm tellin you. The old saying say a fly would slip up on a white shirt and break its neck it would be so slick. All of us could iron. All the girls. We may have just a plain bo'd and we would pad it and put a old white sheet on top of it. Sit it up in the window and have a chair sittin down here. It didn't take us long. It was hard but that's all people knew and it was just as easy then to

14

them as it is now. They paid us such as with a lil money—a lil nothin. When I say a lil nothin you believe it.

The house that we was livin in was on the premises when it was given to my daddy by my grandfather. It was a big house. A great big hall was right straight down all the way down through the middle. On this side was the boys' rooms. Two rooms for the boys. Double beds in each one. Below the boys' rooms was the kitchen and the dinin room. We had a kitchen and dinin. On the front end next the boys' rooms was the guest room. We had a guest room. Nobody never slep in it unless we had guests. Usually be the preacher or anybody else come to spend the night like chil'rens or relatives. Whoever. There was a guest bedroom. We had a bed in there and several chairs and a dresser and there was a o'gan. You have to pedal them o'gans. I was too little to sit. I couldn't pedal. My mother know how to play it. My mother know how to play those acco'dions. And then we had a tall old Victrola that played records. You would call it a livin room and a bedroom combined. When the boyfriends would come to see us that's where we sit in there. They would come co'tin there. On the other side of the house was Mother and Daddy's room and the girls' room below that. The girls' room was a big room with fo beds in it. In the country in those days that's the way they did it where there was a bunch a girls. One big room with fo beds in it. We had a long front po'ch that went all the way across the house. Beautiful flowers we had sittin alongside the po'ch. It was white. Naturally they didn't keep it up like they would now. Then in the country they didn't have grass that you had to cut the yard. They kep it swept. Cleaned and swept. They'd sweep it and it would just be beautiful. Great big yard. And then at the end of the hall goin down the hall my daddy dug a well there so that we had water right there. Right at the step. You could stand on the back po'ch and draw yo water out of the well instead of gettin on the ground. That's the way ours was.

We had two wells. One out in the backyard and one right at the step at the back po'ch. That one out in the backyard is the one they would use for all that washin. No runnin water, no pumps. Not even pumps. We didn't have a sink. Big dishpans that we would wash dishes in one and rinse in another. Dad meant to put a pump in that one he built right at the po'ch and have runnin water but he just never did get to that. The old well had fresh water. It was deeper. The older well was deeper. It had better water. It always tasted better to me. We had an outhouse as well. And all at the same time we had under the shed a buggy, a surrey, and a wagon. At that time Daddy had gotten us a buggy and surrey and a red wagon. A beautiful red wagon. To an automobile. The first car my daddy bought was a 1921 Fo'd. We had a T model Fo'd. That's the biggest Fo'd that Fo'd had then. I think he bought it up at Linden, Alabama. I believe in that area. County seat. I'm thinkin that's where he got it from. And then from hereafter we always kep one. Once we was with a car we was never without a car. Even durin the Depression we had a car. I'm just tellin you what's a fact. It wasn't a fact for most people. But I cain't deny myself of who I am just because a lot a the rest of em didn't have that.

We lived a happy, comfortable life to be right outa slavery times. I didn't know nothin else but the farm so it was happy and we was happy and we could see ourselves a lot mo fo'tunate than the rest of em. We couldn't do anything else but be happy. We accept the days as they come and as they were. Day by day until you couldn't say there was any great hard time. We overlooked it. We didn't think nothin about it. We just went along. We had what it takes to make a good livin and go about it.

The Depression depressed us like it did everybody else but we were survivin real good without knowin the sufferin part about it. Without knowin the real sufferin part about it. We always have made our livin on our property. The Depression was for money. We needed money only to survive through the winter with clothes and what we couldn't not buy to carry us through till the next time it's time to make another crop. So as I say, all that Depression wasn't paid too much attention to. We just managed and went through it. I cain't remember sayin we didn't have no bread and we didn't know where the next bread was comin from. We wasn't naked. We didn't have a whole lot a fancy clothes, but we was not naked. The Depression didn't depress us to that point. We didn't have a whole lot a money in the beginnin but we did have a decent, intelligent, fine livin and everything that went along with it so to make a person happy without sufferin for money or food. Some people didn't know where their next piece of bread was coming from cause they were sharecroppin and when they got through sharecroppin they didn't have but just that much. And just that much don't last but just that lil length of time. Now that's what I call depression. For food, for clothes. We didn't have that to deal with, only people that was less fo'tunate than we was.

I can remember when durin times like that, Dad sold mo cows. And you know what? That didn't dawn on me at the time a Depression. Now I'm just figurin it in. That was part of the Depression. He did that to get money to suppo't us and to carry on like he needed to. Because once upon a time we had too much on hand. What I mean by that is too many cows. There was about fo mules and one ho'se. A whole lot full of cows, calves, goats, chickens. And so when the Depression comes we had enough to sell part of it to carry the situation on. So much so that we never had to sharecrop. We never had to sharecrop for nobody. We was not pulled under. You know we wasn't pulled under when we still got the same property now. It's up there. Everybody got their own part a share. I got mine right now.

The others, they was livin where they could. It wasn't their house half the time. They was livin in Uncle Tom's house and it wasn't fixed up. They was just so lucky through all that. It was colder then up in Marengo County than it usually be now. And it was colder then with all them cracks in them houses. Just had a wall and that was all with the cracks. God took care of em. He did. A lot a times they had to take Sears, Roebuck catalog and tear out every sheet and glue it to stop the holes and the wind from comin in. They had to take flour and make paste and glue up them long holes where the openin was like that apart. But they lived in there. They had babies in there in the cold wintertime and they had nothin but that deep open fireplace. They lived. They sure did. God took care of em. God just have blessed the whole world to come on up from that. After so long there was a few blacks that worked up enough to buy a lil land. Build em a house and enough to work themselves, make them some cotton and co'n. And start growin from there. I don't say they had as much as us but they done pretty good.

We had some resent after Dad started buyin the co'n but it wasn't so much that we didn't get along with em. We stayed humble. We didn't get outhead. None of us. Mother woulda torn us up if she thought we was. "Stay down, stay lil, stay humble, and serve God. That's where yo blessin's come from." We all took that as she told us and we lived like that. We shared with everybody. My mother would 'vide what she had. She was not go'n let a child go hungry. "I got to share this and we got to do this to help Mrs. So-and-So. Her chil'rens goin hungry."

I cain't recall at all the white people resentin our family because we were well off. Not at all. They loved Len Rodgers. That's my daddy. They loved Martha Rodgers. They always took them as people. I cain't remember any white man tryin to cheat or deceive us. Now it coulda been. But if it was I didn't know nothin about it. Mother did washin for so many of em they all met us with nice happy faces. In the quarter to get all this washin they would always wave, the chil'rens. Plenty of em they always waved at us. They hollered at us and we waved at them. Sometime they would use this word which I took for granted not to let that word get to me. "Hey, nigger." You see they didn't know yo name. "Hey, nigger." Well that's bein friendly. That's all they knew. That what they was taught. Indeed I did not take it wrong. I just lived with it. They didn't know to say "Hey, Onnie." That meant the same thing. "Hey, nigger." Cause they all knew us from seein us in the quarter, pickin up clothes, bringin back clothes. My daddy workin here in the house right next do' to em. We got Daddy his dinner in the middle of the day. We met em that way. I got nothin in my heart but love for no human bein under God's sun. From whence I could remember on. I cain't remember a single time that I said I don't like that girl cause she's a white girl. I just cain't remember a single time.

Now you take my mother was havin chil'rens and her neighbor, white woman, if she wanted to go to town to Sweet Water to shop or whatnot, my mother would go up there and nurse that baby. And if Mother had to be gone on a delivery or up there in the town, her baby was carried up there to that white lady. And she fed it from her breast. Fed my mother's black baby from her white breast. They both did that. It was understood. My mother nursed her baby and she nursed my mother's baby. I tell you, Daddy was sent on up to Linden to sit on a jury where you think he was the onliest black that was o'dered in there for years. I remember him talkin about it he did. He was o'dered up there several times. Maybe because my father looked mo like a Indian than he looked like a black man.

You see we had a start but we was honorable. We didn't act like a lot a people woulda acted. We stand down to earth like we supposed to and we had a great big happy smile for everybody, both white and black, and that carry you a long ways. That's the way Mother and Daddy raised us and that's the way we did it. We was raised honorable, carin and sharing. The rest of em wasn't raised like that. We didn't act like we was the big head. We was raised to love, share and give for our family as well as anybody else. And then that's where your progress be come in. You know when you do that God will bless you.

* * *

All down through the years with my mother I was raised religiously. I really didn't know no other way. I didn't want to know no other way in fact. I just come up like my mother raised me and it's still there. They would teach us how to be. In the country we didn't have church that often. Every Sunday but no evenin's through the week because we didn't have lights. We had to use lamp lights—light blue things that hang on the wall. But then finally when I was a big girl we got gas kind that used a pump. My daddy'd pump air in it and then light it and they'd burn like an electric lamp. Had two or three. But that come along later. We had a beautiful service because that was all I knowed. That's the way I knew it so I enjoyed it like that. If it was any different anywhere else I didn't know about that. I only enjoyed what I got. We didn't know no better than to want just what we got.

That day we would get up and get our breakfast and we would go to Sunday school. Then we'd have church worship about eleven o'clock. We had special clothes for church. Might not a been but two or three cause such a big family but had them and we had them clean. In those days there wasn't nothin but just plain cotton anyway. We could wash, starch, light starch em, and iron em and they looked good. I wouldn't want any better. I couldn't get any better. I didn't know any better. So it was fine.

In those days people had home prayer meetin's. Family prayer meetin's. We'll get the Bible. We'll sing a lil church song and then we'll read the Scripture and Mother will explain that Scripture or Daddy the best he could or they would ask us what did we get out of it. Did we understand anything about what they was sayin? And then we would talk and tell how much we didn't understand and to the best of their knowledge they explained it to us. They didn't have as much knowledge of readin like I am right now. But in the sight a God, they was just as much religious as anybody. So that's durin the weeknights. That's Tuesday night and Wednesday night and Friday night that we had prayer meetin's and if we didn't have a full prayer meetin, we studied hard on our Sunday school lesson together and explained.

We usually have whatcha call a revival once a year. We'd at least have service then every day. We would have ten o'clock service. Then we'll have three, fo o'clock service. Then we'll go home. That usually run about a week. That was durin when people had been whatcha call laid by their crops. They had made it and had given it a chance to make itself—you know— get dry. Then we had service from one church to another in the neighborhood. We were baptized merged in the water. It was outside down in the creek. They would clean all the trash from around this beautiful place and it was down in the creek not far from the church. You had to get all the way under. I had on clothes that I wore to church plus I had—my mother would make us a long gown outa yellow mesh, somethin like folks used to make cheesecloth out of. We had a long dress made outa that and then if you go in the water, if you didn't tie a string around it, it would come up, so all the girls would have to tie this string around their dresses. They had to walk slow cause they couldn't make long steps on down in the water. The deacons would lead em there and the preacher would be already in there. He would catch their hands and bring em on down and turn around and baptize em.

I got to be treasurer of the Sunbeam Band. That's the lil group. We'd have meetin's and Mother and the other ladies teached us how to conduct our meetin's and what we should do and what we shouldn't do. So finally when I musta been about thirteen or fo'teen they made me treasurer of the lil Sunbeam Band. My mother was treasurer then of her mission so that rocked on. I took good care of that and my mother helped me with the money. Naturally, what lil bit it was we would carry home and Mother had a big cedar chest she would put hers in one co'ner and mine in the other and lock it. When we went to the meetin we would carry it with us.

So finally my mother taken sick and died. She couldn't talk for about a week after she was struck with that stroke. She couldn't talk for weeks so God blessed her and returned her speech enough that she could tell all us what she wanted done. She said, "Onnie? I tell you what I want you to do. I want you to open that cedar chest." And I did. She said, "Get my money out, it belong to the mission. Count." I counted it up and she says, "Now look on the book and see if that's what's on the book." And it was. That was on the book. She said, "Okay, wrap that up and put it in that big sack and put it back." Then she said, "Get yo's outa there, yo Sunbeam Band money and count it up and see if that's what it tell what we have on the book." It did. She said, "Put that in the sack." She had a lil flour sack then she kep everything in. Hers in one sack and mine in another. And she said, "Put it back. Now come next Saturday when they have the meetin, I want Ada to go with you. You take all this money. You take mine and you turn in yo's cause Mother ain't go'n be here to he'p you keep up with it no mo'."

So I did. I thought about that when she died. She was dead and buried when the time come for me to carry it in. Tied up just like she told me tie it. See Mother made those steps those footprints for me—for us. She made those footprints and you know what? I ain't got no better sense than to walk in them footprints now and I'm afraid not to walk in them footprints. So that's the way my religion comes upon me.

It was a big family of us. Sixteen of us and fifteen got grown. Daddy and Mother had chil'ren one right behind the other. Those chil'rens was raised. Let me put it like that. They wasn't partly raised. As the old sayin goes, we might not a had but one or two dresses, but Mother made us wash them dresses at night and we went clean.

Harvey was the oldest brother. That's the one that lived to got six years old and then got burned and died. Mother was washin and he was putting wood around the pot. In those days they boiled the clothes. He was putting wood around and his clothes got on fire one evenin in March and he died that night. That was a job they never did get a doctor to. Never called the doctor. That wasn't the way you did back then. Mother done the best she could. She taken animal fat, hog lard, and greased a piece a sheet real good cause his clothes almost got burned off a him and wrapped him up in it. But he died. That's what they tell me. I wasn't here. Then in that time in the country people could holler and the person two or three miles away could hear you. That's the way they called for distress and for sick and help. That's what Mother did for Daddy to get Daddy. He was out in the field. Two chil'rens at that time. Two boys. Seem like to me the baby which was my brother Elmer, she had him sittin on a barrel out there when it happened. Mother told me about it. She would always tell it among the chil'rens what happened to their older brother.

Then there was Elmer. That's a good boy. He was the best. He lived to gotten grown and married. He had three chil'ren. My daddy built him a house up above him on the property when he got married. The flu that went through durin World War I that killed so many people got him. That got Elmer. I really don't know how old he was but he was married and had three chil'ren. I was a lil girl when he got married. I could remember. He was workin for that sawmill. He sawed logs. He always sawed logs wherever the company was buyin timber. Mr. Miller and Mr. Cox would buy the timber off this man's land. Their hired hands was hired to go there to saw those lil trees down. Saw up them big long longs. Saw logs to haul to the mill. That was Elmer. But he also had a farm too. Beautiful ho'se, I never will forget that. A ridin ho'se. He liked to ride and I liked to see him ride. Lil girl but I loved to see him comin down the road ridin. He was good. I spent the night with them a many night. He loved me. I was his favorite lil sister.

Now he was the one when my sister-in-law was havin the babies we used to peek through the crack. That was his wife. I musta been around nine. About nine at the time. I can remember things that happened then. My mother would have killed me if she would have known. Mother would never let us in. I went there so I could be with the chil'ren. The other two smaller chil'rens, the two lil girls Elmer had. I was like the nurse for the two lil girls. My mother was deliverin the baby. We were in the other room in the bed, and me, lil nosy, go'n get up and peek through the crack. The two lil girls was in the bed asleep. She delivered on the flo. It was cold that night. Had her on the flo. Her pallet was right across from the fireplace. Big fireplace. I never will forget that. I didn't actually see the baby born but when the baby cried I saw Mother pick it up and cut the cord. There was Charlie. That was the baby boy. Me peekin through the crack.

My sister-in-law, she stayed around awhile after Elmer died. Finally she went to Birmingham. She eventually come back and got the chil'rens. Kep em about a month or two to see that she couldn't handle em and didn't want em. She just didn't want to take time to handle em. She brought em back to Mother and Daddy and they was raised up there with their three last chil'rens. They raised em. Onnie, Lizzie, and Charlie was raised right there with my younger sisters and brothers. Mother and Daddy raised em. I don't know how they felt about that cause they didn't talk that to us with us bein that young. We didn't know what they thought or what they was thinkin. We was cut out of a lot a knowin and sometimes I think that's best.

Curtis was the next one. Curtis was the one that loved his ox. My daddy raised him a set of ox. Built him a wagon. Sawed down the big oak tree, then sawed the wheels, then bolt the holes and made the wagon out of it for his ox. Curtis was drafted. My brother Curtis went to fight in World War I. I can remember my brother Elmer dying when Curtis was in the army. My mother just cried when Curtis went and my brother Elmer died. I can just hear Mother now when I was a lil girl. "When he gets home, Curtis will never see his brother ever no mo." I can just hear that. And she's just sobbin. Made me cry too.

Finally after comin outa the army Curtis got married and had a house. When he came back he went right back to loggin as they call it for the company with his ox. Daddy always would raise him and save him some ox. He lived in the woods with em. Tented in the woods where he fed his ox. When he quit workin he would cook his breakfast or cook his dinner on the fire and feed his ox. Get in his lil tent and go to bed. He loved that. He kep his wife and chil'rens at the house but five or fo days his work was in the woods. He didn't come home. He lived in his lil tent. That was his job. He would carry his food out there. Canned food. Naturally they didn't have ice. For breakfast he would have pancakes and open him a can of sausage. Then he'd cook rice. Whatever he wanted. He was his own boss. You know Elmer was the one hired to go saw those trees down. Then there was my brother Curtis and his ox would split those logs, stack those logs, hook those logs to his ox and drag em out for the trucks to come and get to bring back to the mill. Go into places where the trucks couldn't go. They couldn't go all the way down in them woods. That's what he was doin. He was workin for the company just like Elmer.

Amos was the oddball. There's gonna be a black sheep. He was the oddball. He was the black sheep. They was all Mama's and Daddy's fine boys. All but Amos. He wasn't bad. There was not a mean streak in him. He was just a lil off from the family. In Sweet Water then they had one or two trains that come in haulin logs to that mill. Amos was the fireman. He fired that locomotive. Amos was the one that didn't stand back off white people. He didn't bother em but "don't bother me." He wasn't like the general run of the colored people was that was afraid. Amos was not afraid. He didn't bother em. He didn't pick at em and he didn't cause arouse but just don't bother me. I can remember they just didn't bother him.

I can remember they fired him off that train for some reason. Don't ask me for what reason cause I don't have that answer. He felt like he was treated wrong and they was go'n beat him up like Ku Klux Klans. He got off the train. He come home. He took him a bath. He changed his clothes. They had said what they was go'n do to him. He didn't tell Mother. He didn't tell nobody. He come and took his bath and put all his

28

shells in his pocket and took his shotgun and went back down there and sit down in that quarter as long as he wanted.

Down in that quarter, that sawmill quarter where they was bringin the logs into, there was a lil sto. A commissary sto, a grocery sto, and it had these benches on the po'ch you could sit around on. The ones that own all a that was the ones talkin about hurtin him.

He come home. He got his shotgun and he went back down there. He sat down there with that shotgun across his lap until way after dark. Nobody didn't say nothin to Amos. Amos didn't say nothin to nobody. Amos got up and come on back home and went to bed. He didn't never try to go back to work there. In a day or two Amos lef and came to Mobile right after the episode. But they never did try to bother him. All we know is he stood up to em. So he came on down to Mobile and we didn't hear from Amos for years and years and years. He was the one that seemingly didn't care nothin about family. You know he loved all his family but he just didn't stay around that much. So finally after so many years he come back home. He didn't stay very long. He left and went out in some part of Mississippi and stayed out there. We didn't hear from him for so long. We got the news that said he had killed a woman. He cut her. It wasn't his wife but it was his old lady. He had a wife in Sweet Water. They had built him a house on the place and he had a wife and one son in Sweet Water. He left them to go to Mobile after the episode. He was in his thirties then. I don't know what happened to him. They put him in jail. Some say they attempted to hang him and he wouldn't be taken that morning. So they had to shoot and shot him. Now that's what we heard.

You know Mississippi was death on Negroes in those days. I mean they were bad. If you was a Negro you would do better to be anywhere *but* Mississippi. You better *not* be in Mississippi. Everybody knew how bad it was in Mississippi. To my idea they was much worse in Mississippi. The white people against Negroes was much worse in Mississippi once upon a time than they was in Alabama. News get around. It was all over everywhere. Everybody knew that. We really don't know what become of Amos. Those words hadn't been sent to Mother and Daddy or none a the family but that is what we heard. Somethin happened to him. He never did come back no mo. He was that child you couldn't reach. Mama and Daddy couldn't reach him. He just grew up in his mind "I'm go'n do what Amos want to do" and he did. He wasn't bad. He just drew away. He lifted himself away from the family. Daddy raised his boy when he left right along with Charlie and Lizzie.

My sister Ada is after Amos. Ada was the oldest girl who didn't get to go to school hardly at all. The older chil'rens hadn't much trainin at all. She was such a good girl goin to church all the time and after Mother died she taken care of Dad and she taken care of all of us. She was just a mother. She had boyfriends in her early twenties. Nobody that wanted to marry her but she did have boyfriends. Finally she just let em go by. She was an old maid. Sweet old maid. She was an old maid a long time and so finally one a the deacons of our church, his wife died and he started to likin into Ada. She was way up in her fifties and she just thought it was the wonderfulest thing. He married Ada about three years later. James Adams. He already had his. Already had a big plantation at that time.

That was my brother-in-law that was midwife. It come about this way. When his wife was alive he had so many chil'rens. Bop, bop, bop, bop, bop. His brother bop, bop, bop, bop, bop. Then the chil'rens come on. His older chil'rens. He got tired of tryin to get midwives to deliver chil'rens so he went to the Bo'd a Health and they straightened him up and give him his license. He did it until he was too old to do it. I'm not kiddin. He delivered his own chil'rens' babies, his own babies, his brother's wife's babies in the family and then everybody else that called. Ada never had any chil'ren. I tell you one reason I think Ada was old maid so long. Mother on her deathbed when God returned her speech told each of us what we were to do. She told Ada "you're the mother now" and to my mind Ada took that to heart just like the rest of us did what Mother told us to do. When she got married she was happy to get married.

Ida was the next one. None of em didn't have a chance to get much education. Those older ones especially in those days. Ida married and she had five chil'rens. Ida's husband worked at that sawmill. Ida and the chil'rens had a lil crop workin the farm around and helpin Dad with Dad's crop. That was Ida.

The next was Nettie. Went to school as much as you could expect. Got married. Nettie got married and had fo chil'rens. Married him after he come back from World War I. He come home sick from bein in service. He wasn't able to do very much durin that time but he did work a lil crop and drew a check the whole time. He died about five or six years ago.

Then there was Laura. All the girls went through pretty near the same procedure. She had fo chil'rens. Three boys and a girl. Her husband worked at that mill and then they moved to Bessemer. He worked with the Purina Company. That was Laura.

Betty was the chubby one. Had six chil'rens.

Then there's Sid. Lummy and Sid and J.B. actually worked in the mill. Sid was what you call planer. There's some that saws the lumber and leaves it rough and then there's some that planes it and makes it smooth. Sid made the lumber smooth. That was his job. Sid was easygoin, calm, scary, run in a minute. But he would sure get his in and then run. Down at the quarter they kep pickin at him and kickin him around there. The Klans got after em. No reason. They didn't have to have no reason. Because they was Negroes. Those boys Sid and Lummy had gotten big enough that they could drive around that automobile. They drove it down—there was a great big feed and lawn company where those white boys was workin at. Sid would poke fun. He'll get a lick in and run if he could. But now Lummy would put up a fight. He was different.

Now Sid and Lummy they get after one night right after they got off work. Usually in the wintertime it's dark when six o'clock come when they get off work. Those Klans wouldn't come straight out in the broad daylight and did those things like that. They would wait till they was gettin off work cause they wasn't go'n run a black off his work naturally. Slave labor you know they call it. Because two-thirds of em owned that sawmill. Had a part in it. My brothers I think maybe they heard some lil words on the job because they ran comin home. Sid run and Lummy run different ways. Sid was cryin and callin. Cry quick. Big boy in his teens. If he thought somebody had him in a co'ner.

Sid married, hadn't been long married. Livin just below on Daddy's place they built him a house. He had a lot, his ho'se, pigs, cows, and all. He run home and run on into the house. My sister-in-law said, "What's the matter with you?" He blew the lamp out. They were usin lamp lights then. No electric lights at that time. In those days they didn't have any electricity yet. Blacks nor whites. The power company hadn't made it down that far yet. He blew the lamp out. "Don't say nothin and keep the door locked." Sid got him his gun. Sid was the coward. He was the only one my mother was worried about. Now he would fight to get himself outa somethin. But as soon as he was out, he would run faster than a striped ape. So my mother worried when he got grown he couldn't take care of himself. She got him a shotgun. Not any of the others did she do that for. Not Lummy, not Amos. Sid. And that was the very same gun he used against these men. The very same gun he left behind him when he died. He got the gun and went back out there to the hog pen and got up under his crib where he kep all his co'n. Right after he hid these Klansmen got after him. They're comin up the street creepin and runnin and talkin. Pow, pow, pow, pow, pow. Scared em to death. They left. They didn't bother him no mo. He wasn't shootin to hit at em. He was shootin to let em know what will come next if you run me.

He ran home. The early part of one Saturday night just as dark. He ran home and run on in the house and told his wife to blow out the lamps and get on the flo. He went back out to the lot and got up under his crib in the dark. Here come them comin up the street. One carload and then the rest of em was walkin and callin out to him. Just about the time they got right along that crib he turns that fire. Wasn't shootin for to hit nobody. He said he coulda shot every one of em if he wanted to. "I wasn't shootin at em but they ran." They ran cause they didn't know where it was comin from. I believe he said there was five and one of em was a good friend that he loved so well and who pretended to love Sid so well. They were in their white robes but they didn't have their masks on. A couple of the boss mens didn't want him to know they was involved cause they were so nice to him and he was so nice to them. They were involved in the Ku Klux Klans. I don't know really whether they meant to hurt him or just scare him. The next day the boss men down at the mill said, "You sure did scare the life outa us last night." They didn't bother him no mo. They just had a knack "well we're go'n get after this one this night. We're go'n do this on this night." In those days you didn't know what they would do to you. You couldn't be sure. They might do anything. They might bust in yo house. They might bust into you. They might even kill you. You couldn't know. That was their Saturday night. Sid didn't have any mo trouble. He worked there until they tore that mill down.

Lummy was a branch off Amos. Sid was the mother child. He'd run in a minute scared. He'd run in a minute. But now don't give him a chance to get a lick in and run, he do that.

Lummy was different. Lummy ain't go'n dodge. He get you face to face. In those days time had ruled and we could have church parties and school parties. Young people would get together at one another's house or in the yard and make a big fire and then have fun parchin peanuts. They had lil Friday night parties and lil Saturday night parties. They didn't have nothin else to do. Nowhere else to go. There was nothin to drink. In those days people made, I would say shinny. Only the homemade moonshine that they call it. Those is what you call the good ole days but they was bad ole days. They couldn't have a good party without these white boys would show up. Two Bradley boys. White boys pickin at the black. Whenever them black folks would have a party them two boys would go. Take advantage of black girls and all such as that.

When Lummy got to be eighteen years old he broke that up. They was havin a great big cookout in the woods and them two Bradley boys showed up. Lummy got into em. He tore em up at that time. He whipped those boys. It was a fight, honey. It was a fight. Lummy tore that fire all to pieces with them boys. Them boys flew when they got loose from Lummy. Believe me they run. We didn't have no mo trouble with them. Never did hear no mo about it. Never heard no mo about it. I was afraid for a long time. They never did let Mother and Daddy know it. They knowed what they'd got—torn up. We knew. Sid told us. Whispered around and told us, my brother Sid. He ain't go'n stay there and help Lummy do it. He run off in the dark and watch.

Lummy never had any other trouble with white folks. One reason he didn't. He tend to his business. I give them boys credit. They tend to their business. Whenever they got into anything if it was anything they got into it was them white pickin at black. Lummy lived there for years after that. Thank God nothin happened. He worked at that sawmill until he left Sweet Water.

The next was Lily Mae. She had one son. In fact she miscarried a couple a chil'ren. She had one son and she taken pneumonia and died. He was seven months old. The next sister, Evie Louise, raised the seven month-old baby along with her baby. He was older than Lily Mae's baby. Evie taken Lily Mae's baby and raised it. Then Onnie was next to Evie Louise. I was the fo'teenth child. Next to Onnie is Bernice. Bernice got married and her and her husband had a pressin cleaners. They had a business up in Sweet Water. Finally they moved to Mobile and brought the business here in Prichard. They had three chil'ren. They're all three here in Mobile. Then there's J.B., the baby.

In those days black folks wasn't gettin much education. We went to school on a sho't term. We had five months, Negroes did, in those days, to go to school and we didn't went sometime half a that. That's all they would allows. That's all the white people allowed us to have. There was so many of us and then there wasn't any money and they made us pay a lil fee for every child durin that time. When there wasn't no money to live on. You wouldn't want to believe it with things the way they are now. I don't know whether they were makin white people pay at that time or not. But we had to pay and then we had to buy our own books. The books had to be bought. We all went to school in my family for a certain length of time the best we could. None a the older ones didn't have a chance to get much education. They had to do everything there was to do. They plowed, they hoed. When the time come in the spring a the year, naturally they make preparations for farmin. That's in order to clean up the old co'nstalks and whatnot from last year. They had all that to get up. None of us got the full education that we shoulda gotten.

The school I went to was an all-black school. There wasn't very many good schools. There wasn't very many teachers. Then there was one lil schoolroom that taught about ten or twelve classes in that one room. Sometimes just one teacher and then it was two and then after so long all the fifth and sixth grade students will help teach the primary grades. I often thinks about that a lot a times but thank God we made it. We made it through. I'm talkin about the Negro race.

I was about eight years old when I started school. In those days you didn't start at the age of six. I had ten years of school when I was growin up. I was gettin ready to go to high school when Mother taken sick and died. Cause high school wasn't up in Sweet Water. We had to come to Thomasville. That woulda been grades eleven and twelve.

In Sweet Water goin to school none a the streets was paved, none a the roads that was roads then was paved. We had to walk it or Daddy—if it was rainin and sloppy too much— Daddy carried us in his wagon cause it was too many of us to ride in the car. So he would carry us in the wagon. And when it's pretty sunshine and we come back and the whites was ridin in the school buses and throwin out the windows, we would have to get way out so they couldn't throw rocks and bottles and whatnot that they had in there to hit us with. Get out of the way. That's what Mother taught you—get out the way. Don't fight back as long as they don't hit you and don't hurt you—get out of the way. That's what she said and we accept that and we did that. Not only us. All the Negroes. They called us nigger. That's it—plain nigger. That was the word they used. And you know what? They didn't try to learn any better in those days. They thought that word fitted our black face and they enjoyed usin it and that's the way it was. And they'd use it as a dirty slang.

Now the black man, the black person had a hard way to go. Was treated bad in those days. But God took care of em. He did not budge one consent. He didn't let man destroy em. You know what I mean by man? He didn't destroy em, but he gave em a hard way to go. You know usually in those days the white person didn't care too much about Negroes as a whole. They went as a mob group in those days. Then they went from the mob to that Ku Klux Klan. Even if they didn't in the name then of the Klan, they went in the name of the white people. Same thing. It was the po white people. Not the real good white people was no involved in doin's like that. Common kind was involved. We knew they was a gang of white people that would get themselves together livin in pure evilness and they would beat up black people but they didn't bother white people. It's a gang gettin together callin themselves the Ku Klux Klan. That's what they were. I knew all about the white robes. I heard about that.

I can remember Mother teachin and tellin us about that when we were young. She said they disguise themselves with the hooded caps and the white robes. Like white sheets they would have on and they would beat up black folks. Mother's sittin down teachin us that and she said don't get revenge. She would always tell us in those days if you meet a bunch of white chil'rens comin from school, go around em. Don't meet em. Pass around em like that. Give em the road. She told us not to fight back. All the time Mother told us to beware of em. My daddy told my brothers not to fight back—run. Get home. We paid attention other than the oddball Amos.

Everybody know to shy the Klan when I was growin up. They were rough because people would talk about it. Things like you have to be careful because in those days they didn't know nothin else to do but be careful and run. They couldn't fight back. There was a lot a happenin's. They would run em and catch em and beat em and kill em, some of em and leave some of em half dead. I'm sure they were the ones doin a lot a the castrations. I've heard of lynchin. I really don't know of any certain person but I've heard a lot of it—that lynchin they did. It happens wherever Negroes was and you know they was everywhere after slavery time. They were everywhere. Then they got to the place that they didn't lynch but they would castrate him and leave him. There was a lot a castrations.

There was—I never will fo'get—there was a man we call Mr. Frank, and he really was from slavery time, lived by himself. They beat him up bad. They even castrated him. I'm just lookin at this lil sho't, fat man. You know when you do a man like that, he usually get fat. They do. Even a woman have a hysterectomy usually get fat. Hardly got any control over it. You will gain mo weight than usual. And I'm lookin at this man right now when I was quite a young girl, how fat and chubby he got. You know a sho't, fat man. After they did him like that. I don't care how hot it was, he wore his overcoat. They did that a lot, honey. They did that a lot. I had a couple of cousins to be castrated. It didn't cause that much stir cause the black people was always the underdog anyway. The white knew wasn't nothin go'n be done about it.

Now I tell you what they would mostly do. If they thought a black man was after a white woman, was likin into a white woman, off go his head and his foots too. Now that's when they did it. They did it then. More frequently than any other time. That happened, honey. That's just the way it was. But now let me tell you one thing. In those days—you might not like this what I'm fixin to say now. In those days when the white woman was involved, the white woman mostly involved herself. I know that those Negro mens was afraid to do better. Black men was really afraid to even think of rape. Along in these days black mens taken a notion to rape a white woman just like they would me.

Dr. Jones from Sweet Water delivered a baby for a white woman. When the baby were born Dr. Jones says, "This is a goddamned black nigger baby." Everybody knew that's what the doctor said from the black girl was there workin at the time.

40

I was a lil baby pickin up clothes in the mill quarter and that's where she was livin. They were all usin heaters and fireplaces then. Mostly heaters—no gas, no nothin like that. This particular black man would carry wood that was sawed from the lumber, the ends of the lumber, to these houses. These white houses in the quarter so they can have wood to burn in the wintertime. He was attached to the situation. That's how it come about him gettin the white lady pregnant. Indeed if it was him it was her idea is what I'm gettin at, durin carryin that wood. Ain't nobody to know if it actually was him or not that did it. He was the likeliest one to attach, you see. That's all.

He had to leave. I don't know what come of him. I cain't remember him ever comin back. He knew the Ku Klux would get after him. If they got their hands on him that woulda been it. If somethin occur among the black and the white, the black knew they were go'n get it. As the old sayin goes, "Skip city." They knew how to leave. "I'm go'n settle for leavin cause the mob was after for to kill me." They go away. They had a pretty good easy way of gettin away. The barges and boats goin down to Mobile come from down the Tombigbee River. They'd catch those barges down on the other side. A lil place on the other side Sweet Water called Nanafalia. Not far from there is the river. We see'd a lot a that. And then freight trains that was runnin. You know how they hold on freight trains. They are known to ride between all the logs that they was haulin, whatever they was haulin, an empty boxcar and all. The best way that they could get outa there. It used to occur a lot a times. I just heard about well the mob as they would used to call em was after So-and-So and he got away. I could hear the grown people talkin about it. That's the way it happened all the time and I never could question them about it. Not too much. They didn't allow chil'rens to dictate in. So that kep me down a lot but I knew that's the way it was. And I knew when it happened and the time it happened because I could hear.

That baby was the cutest lil thing. My mother's half sister was who was workin there. They gave it to her after so many months. Cutest lil thing you ever seen. You know I think those are the prettiest chil'rens there is, anyway. They are the prettiest chil'rens you'll see, half white and half black. Hardly any of em is kinky head. You know I can tell too cause I've delivered some of em. So they gave the baby to my mother's half sister and she kep that lil girl until she was about six years old. She was married, but she couldn't have kids, didn't have kids. But then he—white lady's husband—couldn't stand knowin that she had it and he went and told where the baby was and what happened. Then the government got a hold to it and come and taken that lil girl away from my aunt. It liked to have killed her.

But now it wasn't always a white woman. That wasn't all the time it. That wasn't the reason all the time. Mainly it was their hatred and their evil heart. There don't be no reason why. They just do it. They take a notion and they do it. They didn't have to accuse em in those days. They didn't have to have a reason. Or they'll make up a reason. Because we was Negroes, that's all I can say. We had to keep to ourselves. I could say a slight word to you and you could say anything in this world to me you wanted to. If I would answer you back I was go'n get it. "That nigger don't sass me. We go'n do this and do that" and

42

they'll wait for the chance together. They were mean and dirty. I'd rather have a black dirty body cause I can clean that up easy, than to have a black dirty heart.

I know this from my parents. This wasn't durin slavery but they still treated em the slave way. This cousin of mine comin outa the field—now I remember this, I was a lil bitty girl when this happened. But I remember him and his lil boy, was older than me, was comin outa the field and he stopped. No paved streets then. He stopped at the main street, he stopped to clear a branch running across the road. And as he stopped up on the hill, these two brothers come up. And I don't know why. I ain't never known the reason why. They didn't have to have no reason. They shot him down by that branch right in front of his lil son. The lil son musta been about seven or eight years old. Shot him down. If they hadn't killed him he woulda drowned. He wasn't able to get up outa the water. Shot him down. The lil boy took the mules and led em on up the road callin for help. Looks like they woulda shot the lil boy but they let him live. I know when that happened. I remember that well. There wasn't nothin my family could do about it. There was nothin that they could say about it or do about it but speak by themselves and cry about it. It was so sad. I went to the funeral. I was a lil girl. Just about the age of that son. And he lives over there by the bridge right now. But this was one a the no'mal things that happened. Those boys in those days—I ain't go'n call their name cause everybody know. You didn't have to have nothin against him except that he was black.

My grandmother was in slavery days. She was a slave on a white plantation. In those days you had nowhere else to live but there. I cain't recall too much about the Civil War. Alls I know is my grandmother was a slave and lived on after the war. My grandmother was partly most in slavery days. It was a whole lot a slavery when my mother was young. I know my mother would say that my grandmother and all there were certain times that they had to go around. They couldn't go through Mr. Charlie's place to get to the lil area over there where the people was livin on the place. They had a lil pig trail they used to go around. You couldn't drive up to the house. They had to drive as far as they could with the buggy or wagon and leave it there and then walk up.

Durin slavery they was pushed to do what they did. They didn't ask em to do it nicely. You know what I'm talkin about. I can just picture that. I've heard so much of it. I can just picture—I can see it right now. But you know what? It doesn't hurt my heart. They would be discussin it and tell how. Not that they revenged, want to get revenge from it. They was just there talkin about it and discussin how it went on and what happened.

I never will fo'get, there was a lady, my father's aunt on his mother's side, said that when she left the house where she was workin at—I fo'get what the man asked her to do and she didn't do it. He knocked her in the head with a club. And she got that lil to'chlight. It was light she got it and she held it up for when she left the house cause she lived across the branch. You know it's like goin through the bushes—a lil path to her house. Good

44

lil ways you know. But they heard her hollerin. She was comin home from fixin supper that night and when she got near the house with that lil light tryin to see her way to come, God let her walk just in the do'. They all opened the do' for her and she fell up in the do' and that's it. Dead from knockin her in the head. And they heard her callin but God kep her on her feet. She fell in the do'. They have told that so much and told that so much, that was just there. Somethin he asked her to do. Lil minor thing. I don't know whether she said somethin. He asked her to do it and she hadn't gotten around to it. She'd forgotten it or somethin like that. I've heard so much.

I can remember hearin this story so many times. This was a man that had worked and plowed all day long. Carried the mules home to give em their supper. They had already had theirs. And then they called him out from his house—a bunch a white people—and he went out the back do' cause he knew that when there was a crowd they'd get up at night like that. Three or fo. They know what it is. They want either to kill him or beat him up. He run and they got behind him and runned him. He went to the field on in and he went runnin in the creek and he drowned himself. And they just left him. Nobody never got him out to bury him or nothin. They was afraid to get him. That's supposed to been an uncle of mine, my mother's brother, who was older than she was.

Out of all that we went along like happy-go-lucky. No ill will in our heart or mind or nothin. We lived like human bein's supposed to live. That hasn't made me resentful at all. I'm glad God kep me. I'm so happy I don't know what else I'd want to do. You know why? It's payin off. Indeed white people have done black people wrong. And you know what? The general run of em know it. They admit it. A lot that won't admit it knows it. But there's plenty of em that admit it. God did not let it deal with me too much and I'm glad cause if you get yo mind set on that you cain't go on to nothin else.

Tradition

Mother tried to give us the best thing to grow up on. She loved to get us around her sittin on the flo around her and she start tellin us these things that would he'p us. She would just sit us round and she'd start tellin us these stories about her mother-in-law that was such a good midwife. That was my grandmother on my daddy's side. My grandmother was a midwife while she was a slave. She did white and black. I don't know whether the wealthy white families. They probably used the doctors. But didn't all of em use the doctors. I know they didn't. They used midwives too. And then she was with my mother for the few older chil'rens. She delivered my mother's. She was with her on the few older chil'rens and then she died. She died a long time ago when my mother was just beginnin to have all her babies.

In Sweet Water I heard so much a big story about my grandmother. That she was such a good midwife and did so much work, nurse work and he'p people in the country from one place to the other when they gotten sick. Befo they could send for the doctor they would send for my grandmother and I heard that over and over again. I could always hear a story about her—the things she did. The older people when they get these conversations goin about that. But mostly my mother. I could remember my mother tellin about how my grandmother would have to get up when they come after her. If she didn't went back with them they would drive the buggy. They'd take the wagon or they'd take the buggy. I know that's the way they did my mother and she told me that's the way they did Grandmother. In the buggy and in the surrey and then on ho'seback too. She was doin both white and black at that time. It was just a lot of experience to me to listen at that. That just got in my mind and just stayed within my mind that that's what I want to do and that's the way I want to be. They said she was always ready to go. When she came in she do the same thing that I do. She repack her bag befo goin to bed. I have to have three bags cause some days I had two babies or three babies in one day. So I couldn't very well go to sleep or lay down and rest without repackin my bag and ready to go.

My grandmother inspired me and it still is in me today. It was just in me to do what I did because if it hadn't I'd a done somethin different. I'd rather see a baby be born in the world than to eat if I'm hungry. I love it. I'm lookin at the work of God that man didn't do and that's somethin to think about and I enjoyed it. My grandmother I think she gotten pneumonia as for her death. Gettin up cold days and nights. They said she caught her death he'pin somebody.

My mother did the same work. My mother delivered a many babies. She had the same record. My mother was not a licensed midwife. They didn't license em then. Sure didn't. She didn't repo't any births. I mean she didn't fill out any birth certificates. If it was white she repo'ted to the doctor that was comin. With white my mother always worked in a place where the doctor was comin. Plenty times she done the work befo the doctor got there. And then along about those days they just didn't repo't all the births anyway. They don't have a record of me at birth nowhere.

Mother got and my daddy too got stricter and harder deliverin babies when they started licensin. Started goin up bein trained. I don't have any idea what time that was when they started doin that. I don't remember the year but I do know hearin my father speak about my mother not bein licensed. He told her that she had to be careful and if she wanted to she had to go ahead and try to get her license. She didn't do that. She was havin chil'rens so frequently and fast herself she didn't have time to even think of licensin as she was workin like she were. But she would go when somebody called her. She was from one place to the other doin deliveries.

I could just see right now my mother workin and goin on delivery. I could see it right now. I can just see when they came for her. I can remember she loved to work the gardens. She would work those gardens and I can remember the man comin for her to ride in that wagon for miles. If the buggy was gone and the boys had the wagon, they'd come for her in their buggy or if he was on a ho'se she would walk for miles. They would come and say, "I come after you. Miss Jane, she fixin to have a baby." Mother just start gettin ready. She'd get on all those long aprons. I don't care how hot it was—you know they wore those long dresses then. Every time I see a granny midwife she be in this form. Her long dress, her long apron, her old coat and lil hat. That's how my mother looked. In those days that's the way since they was a woman. That's the way they wore their clothes since they were women and chil'rens. A wife and mother wore their dresses long always, even in summer. Most women would look like this anyway especially the midwife with them long aprons.

I hear "granny midwife" all the time. That's what it was. That's what it was from the beginnin. My grandmother and mother were called that. They'd call her granny. Many years ago they used to say, "That's yo granny. That's yo grannymother. She delivered you. She was the first one to put her hands on you. She's the one that made you cry, got the breath in you." White and black used to tell em that and they still do now. You can go right now and start talkin to somebody about my age and lil older and quite a bit older. They'll say, "I was delivered by a granny midwife." A black woman, a granny midwife. I was delivered and all my sisters and brothers was. I got a whole lot a grandchil'ren myself. Catchin babies—that's what they call it. They'd say, "Where's Tinny goin?" "She gone to catch So-and-So's baby." That's what they called it.

Mother would go if it's in the night. She would always wake up and carry one of us smaller ones to walk back with her because he would be goin to work when the baby come. She didn't want to do it by herself—walkin. If not be that way my daddy would send one a the grown-up boys the next mornin to go after her. Several times I can remember at night bein waked up as a lil girl when they come for her to ride in that wagon for miles. And I went with Mother to deliver her own grandchil'ren. The older ones used to follow one another just like that havin babies. When we got there naturally they wouldn't let us in the room to see what it's all about. As I have always said, in those days, Mother and them, they didn't let us in on everything. The big happenin's of childbirth and pregnancy.

My mother did not mention to me one time what to do about my period when it started. Nobody to tell you exactly how it is. I didn't know nothin about it. Nobody to tell me nothin about it. Nobody hadn't told me how to take care of myself. I don't know why mothers in those days wouldn't tell you. One a my older sisters give me a hint and I want to show you how clever God made me. Naturally we wouldn't go buy a sanitary pad. There wasn't sanitary pads to be bought. We had to make em. I worried about that day and night. It come to me just as good how to get me a needle and thread and a old piece of—we made slips then outa unbleached mesh. It was new material. Yellow. Had these left. I had been makin slips for everybody. I went in there and got me a piece a that and I made it so it could come around this way. I made it so I could button it. I put a button and a buttonhole on there and I made one piece that I could fasten on back there and brought it through to here and could pin it to hold the piece that I put on it. Nobody hadn't told me. Nobody hadn't told me one iota thing. It come to me and I made it and wrapped it up in a lot a paper and then stuck it up under the house until that time come. Nobody told me one thing. I don't know why. Plenty of mothers just didn't tell you. I guess they were ashamed and that's the way their mother treated them. Mother thought she was right in her own way for not lettin me know that. She put that outa my sight.

Mother told us about interco'se. Now she told that to try to save us. My mother would get us around and she'd sit down and get us around on the flo and relay everything to us. "If you mess around with one a them boys and one a you come up here with a baby I'm go'n kill you. I'm go'n kill you." I believed what she said. I didn't have no better sense than to believe what Mother said. That's the way I am today. Believin what she said. Still doin what she said for me to do. I never let that cross my mind. "You get a baby and I'm go'n kill you." Mother opened up about menstruation after she knew we was menstruating. Then she tell me how to take care of it but I think I had menstruated about three months befo she did. I always tried to look out for myself and it come. Who woulda thought that I would sit down and it come to me exactly how to fix that and then go hide it up under the house wrapped in paper?

So you see I wasn't in the room with my mother while she was deliverin babies. They just wouldn't allow it. Mother would never let us in. But I always was nosy. I would want to know what was goin on. You know me. I peeked through the crack to see what was goin on. I really did. Cause she'd take us with her and leave me in the other room and I just couldn't do that. I'd have to see what was goin on. I wanted to see as much as I could what was goin on and I did that as much as I could. And all that then was just buildin up in me. That put me on the go. That's what I want to be. I want to do that. Sho do. That is what I was livin in my hopes and my prayers. I prayed to God to let me do those kinda things.

Now the midwives in those days—let me tell you abo midwives in those days. When they go on a delivery, they didn't just go on a delivery. They do the cookin and the washin. It wasn't so much of the midwifin. They was there to he'p with anything they could do. He'p with the other smaller chil'rens. My mother wasn't paid hardly anything a lot a times. If she was paid at all they might give her co'n, chicken, greens outa the garden if we didn't have any and such like that. There wasn't any money to pay em.

The midwives would always make them a sack. They didn't have bags naturally like that I have. But they would make them a sack and they would put their stuff in there and put a drawstring on it and draw it. Mother had a great big tall chifforobe. She would put it in there when she wasn't usin it. My mother would get—they used to call it shoestring. They didn't have shoestrings. It was material they would have set aside. You know when you buy material—the end of it. Well she would tear that all the way down and she would cut it in pieces so she could have it to tie the cord with and she would boil it. She had a plain pair of scissors. She had that and she would sterile it.

In those days the doctors didn't tell em what to do. They used the old home remedies, mostly come from the Indian remedies. The midwife then would always carry her herbs that she was goin to make teas out of to give them somethin warm to drink. They made teas outa this and teas outa that and drank it all down through the times. There's a bush in the woods called sassafras and you dig the root out of it, dry it, boil it, and make a tea out of it. I love it. They made a tea outa hen feathers. You would parch the hen feathers and make the tea. And it worked. It worked. Through God it worked.

I'll tell you what they used to do even when they got in labor. It was a big hand on givin em a big dose of castor oil. That would work their bowels off real good and bring the contractions close together. My grandmother did that. They would always use that homemade grease. They didn't have Vaseline but they had animal fat that had been cooked all the water out of. You know they put it on the stove. Even as soon as my daddy would kill a cow my mother would get that tallow and cook it on the stove until it wasn't bubblin at all. All the water is out of it then. That's a good salve. They do pig fat and ho'se fat the same way. They would grease the mother, the vagina, with that.

I could remember they usually put an ax under the bed. Now they did this for what you call the afterpains. They didn't do that when she was having labor pains. Mothers in turn some of em still do have real severe afterpains. Afterpains after the baby comes can be just as hard some of em as pains to deliver the baby. So they put a knife or a ax up under the bed with the blade turned straight up to cut the pains. I could remember even the fever, that fever that they usually have, that afterfever. They usually put a pan a water up under the bed. They said that cools the fever off. If they thought they was go'n have a hemorrhage they had stuff that they made up to give and it worked and did just as good as all this expensive doctor medicine now. That's what they knew in those days. It probably helped in their sight and made them thinkin that was the way to do it. No doctors, no nothin. When I was a lil girl the midwives used all those kinda things because they had nothin else. They had to use somethin so they used what was in their mind and through God it worked.

In those days they didn't use pads that you threw away. They would use in the country you know they had these quilts that they pieced up. The old clothes that we wore and wore out, the skirt part a the dress wasn't hardly tore up. We would take that and cut it into blocks and sew it together to make quilts. We had quilts stacked up like that. Clean. We needed all of em. They would always save those old quilts, raggedy ones, and they would boil em and sterile em. Put em under to protect the bed. Didn't use newspapers and then a small pad like we use now thank goodness. It's sterile. It's sterile when they get through boilin it. The type of water that we wash with is hot. But I'm talkin about boil in them old black pots they got. Outside. Big old pot. And they just push it down and push it down until it boils and boils and boils. And when they get it out there it's sterile and no stains at all. No stains. Then hang it out in that hot sun. They would wash those same old quilts and fold em up and pack em back and use em again. That's the way they did it. I never will forget. You know in the country, honey, they made whatcha call lye soap to wash with. You heard about that. You make soap enough to wash off all the year. You pack it away and wash off it all the year. It was strong.

Usually with the afterbirth they would burn it. That was easily done cause in olden times they either had an old heater or a fireplace that they could wrap it up in paper or rags and put it right in there on that and it would burn it up. They did a good job considerin that's the best of the knowledge in those days.

I never known nobody to die that Mother was involved in. Now I've known babies to die. Half the time I don't know whether they was stillbo'n babies or whether they died bein born or afterwards. What was the cause of death I don't know. Those older people in those days did not talk that to us girls. They didn't talk to us on things like that. They thought we had time enough to learn that. One thing, honey, babies didn't have no mother's care, no vitamins. No such thing as prenatal care then. Weren't hardly any doctors to give it anyway. In those days they would go once or twice. My mother she had those fifteen grown chil'ren. I bet you she didn't go to the doctor two times among the whole fifteen. And then half the time, three fo'ths the time, the mother ain't got enough to feed herself properly. There was quite a few miscarriages in the days that my mother was havin babies. There was mo then than there is now. They had to work so hard. All the pregnant women worked out in the fields. Durin slavery they'd have their baby tonight and get up and go to the field in the mornin. I've heard that so many times.

The white doctors at this time—let me tell you about the white doctors at this time. I don't think they paid too much attention to the black families then, because the spirit of the white people then didn't go out for the black people. They didn't care. They didn't care cause they didn't feel sorry for em.

I don't know whether to say that's the way they thought we supposed to been treated or not but that's the way we was treated and they thought nothin about it. They didn't give it any attention whatsoever. I feel like they thought it was right. One thing, honey, two-thirds of em didn't use the black at that time as a human bein. They thought that we was—as they used to call us—animals. We were like animals. So they didn't have any feelin for us.

And some of em were livin exactly like animals then because they didn't know no better. They didn't have enough money to do nothin. They didn't know no better than to live like animals. Go around for weeks and weeks and weeks and months without a bath. The skin even begin to look like animal it was so dirty. The Negroes at that time didn't meant to be like that. That's all they knew. That's the best two-thirds of em knew. They didn't know how to clean up. You should blame the white folks for not teaching the po ole black person. I think the white person in those days shoulda took mo interest in the Negroes since he hadn't had any schoolin.

They didn't make any effort to he'p the po black people. They didn't send nobody. Nobody wasn't goin out to teach em how to keep clean. All they was lookin from them was to get up and get out and go to work. Get out in the field. Get out. They didn't teach em how to keep clean or be clean or nothin. They *was* filthy. They *was* nasty. But they needed somebody to teach em. They didn't have any better and no way to get any better. He hadn't done anything to learn any better, to know any better, and they didn't try to learn us any better in that time. The doctors didn't fool with it.

I don't know how, we just kep marchin along. When one start to look like he doin better the other start up too. I am a great hand in watchin you do good and I can do as good as you. I have always felt that within me. That's where I was mostly beginnin. And then it start creatin in the black families. "I'll watch you. If you wash yo face I'll wash mine. I'll watch you. If you lace yo shoes I'll lace mine." I feel like that's the way the beginnin of Negro education from copycattin. I know in that time I was a good copycat cause I loved to not let nobody do hardly no mo than I could do.

In that time there was no hospital that they could go to have no baby. They didn't have clinics. They didn't have doctors. A doctor every now and then. When you call one, even if you call one today, he *might* come tomorrow. He *might* come tomorrow. So how could we—I think that's one reason in the sight a God that midwives come about. There was an intention from God because that was God's program for the women to have babies. It was the midwife or nothin.

There was no phone in Sweet Water. They'd have to get on their ho'ses in the wagon or buggy and go get that midwife. There wasn't not only no roads, a lot a times there wasn't nothin but a path that you had to walk through the woods to get to this house over here and that house over there. It was just a path and if you didn't have a lantern light—if you went at night you would have to carry a to'ch. A fat long splinter to'ch lit so you ⎯ ⎯ how to go through that lil path. They wouldn't have waken up a white doctor then, see. They'd been afiₗ that. Cause you know that's when most babies are boₗ night.

You know why the blacks avoided the white doctors? Because, honey, they avoided the whites period. They be afraid to meet em. If a white person comin, they'll go around. To walk way around him to keep from meetin him. You know they didn't want the white people to see their home cause they couldn't do no better at those times. They just couldn't do any better. And then they was treated so bad and so cold by the doctors. The doctors thought the black person was mostly too filthy for him to put his hands on. They talk to em just like they was a dog that didn't have human sense. They did not want that kinda treatment. They didn't deserve that kinda treatment cause they was human beins.

About three or fo miles away from Sweet Water, what you call Nanafalia, Alabama, there was Dr. Clyde. Dr. Jones in Sweet Water and Dr. Clyde in Nanafalia. That's it. That was it. That was not enough to cover. There just wasn't enough doctors. How could those two doctors, one in each place and they was eight and ten miles apart or mo than that from Sweet Water to Nanafalia? And then way over in Cutland was another doctor—cain't think of his name—durin that time. Now that was goin Sweet Water, Nanafalia, and Cutland. Miles apart. Miles. With the place full a farmers. That's all they was doin in those days and you know how many people that was. Great big black population. They lived distance apart. Distance apart. A doctor was impossible for him to keep up with all these cause women was havin babies like cats havin kittens durin these times with no prenatal care whatsoever.

I cain't remember a doctor go in a place in my whole time in the country to deliver a black baby. I don't remember a single doctor not a single time deliverin a black baby at home. Not one. And I cain't remember them callin in a doctor for complications on a delivery. The Lord blessed us so, I was just thinkin, so there wasn't very many complications. It's not nearly as complicated to have a baby and for a baby to live as they say and as they pretend because this is the work of God and God never fails on His work. Those old midwives and the ones that wasn't midwives that knowed how to do the work, they went and did it. Such as my mother. They did that. I don't remember a single doctor deliverin a black baby at home. Not in my whole life. Cause if they sent for him the baby would been there and probably some of em walkin befo he got there.

I remember when my mother had a stroke. Musta been around nine or nine-thirty on a Sunday night when she had that stroke. I never will fo'get—we was havin a prayer meetin and she prayed the last prayer. And when she got up off her knees she had the stroke and we all saw it. And right then and there my daddy got my brother, I don't know which one, got in the car and went to get the doctor for her. For a stroke. And you know when he came? About eleven o'clock the next day. That was at nine o'clock on a Sunday night, and he came the next mornin after his breakfast. Fact is we just couldn't get one over in Sweet Water. Had to go down in Nanafalia to get one. Dr. Jones finally come. Sho did. Not until the next mornin.

Fact a business, a lot a white families years ago did nothin but use midwives. And most midwives at that time was black. They didn't have many white midwives period. But the white race have always used the black midwives. They've always used em. I don't know whether white people just didn't want to be bothered or they didn't like the job or why they didn't do very much of it. And wasn't only white sharecroppers my mother delivered for. There was white people that owned property. You don't call em sharecroppers the ones that own the property.

She helped em. That's the way my mother come in a lot a times—workin with the doctors. There has been a doctor came in and then they're go'n send for my mother too. The doctors mostly time they are there to deliver that baby and get goin. They're not go'n clean up any of it. They will have Mother there with the doctor knowin Mother's go'n do the cleanin up afterwards. This would be white families. Mother would do whatever need to be done. Sometime she would get the house all cleaned up. Mother all settled and baby all settled. See the doctor's not go'n bathe that baby, not go'n dress that baby or nothin like that. That's go'n be the midwife. The doctor would fill out the birth certificate. It happened a lot a times that the baby was born befo the doctor got there. So you see it was white and black alike that used midwives. It was never hard to get a midwife unless she was already on another case. All you had to do was to go down and pick her up.

The people in Sweet Water respected midwives a great deal. Loved all of em. Even my brother-in-law in bein a male midwife. He was respected highly among em. And he was licensed. Very thankful to have him to do that work. There was quite a few midwives but they was distance apart durin the time of my brother-in-law. He'd gotten so old that he had to quit workin. But a lot a times he went and wasn't able to. He began to get old and feeble but he went. He still went. Sho did.

God gave the po, as they say, the ignorant black person, knowledge enough to use home remedies to kill whatever. If they didn't have sense enough through God's power to do that they woulda gotten killed off cause the doctors wasn't comin out. Mostly those remedies come from Indian people. Marengo County was swampy and then the hot sun when workin the field. There was this malaria fever that would rotate around from one person to another. So there was a weed that my mother and all used to get. I don't know if this is the proper name for it or not—jumpsin weed. Now the jumpsin weed is the weed that they laid around em to cool the fever. They would get that and tie it around the head, lay it on the head and tie it around the ear for high fever. They would lay oil on the chest and oil on the stomach for high fever. The jumpsin weed lays cool to the body. Sometimes that fever would be so high until when you take it off you done parched that green leaf up.

Then there's another weed with a lil yellow flower in the top of it. Usually call it bitterweed. Mother would gather that as she would anything else in the summertime and let it dry to make teas through the winter because no doctors. It taste just like quinine. They would give that to em for fever. Most chil'rens come down with high fever for some reason or another especially in the summertime. No doctor that you could take it to. No one to come see you so they would make these teas. I reckon God just put His hands on it and let it work because we had no alternative but use what was in our minds at those times.

Now for a cough, a bad cough, we would use those hog-hoof teas. Now my mother made us use that tea. My daddy killed hogs for our po'k meat all the time and we would save the hoof off the hog feet just like we would anything else for winter teas and salves. They used to use the inside of an eggshell, that lil thin piece. I wished I could remember what they did with that. They used to use that in some kinda tea too.

Instead of Vicks salve—didn't have no money to buy it with nohow—they used the tallow fat from animals. That fat they would boil that down and put a lil turpentine in it. I can remember my mother used to cook it up and put it in a jar and put it up on the shelf among the other vegetables and things so she'd know where it was when it come time to use it. Mostly she used it in the wintertime. She would get a piece of flannel—old wool pants or old wool skirt—and put it on that. Grease that up and lay it on the chest. Or if they wasn't confined to bed they would put it on the chest and tie a lil string around the neck so it would always be right here on the chest. Put it on the chest with a string around the neck so it could absorb some of the cold. Open up the chest from the smell of the turpentine. No doctor—had to have some kinda medicine. It worked. But now since the world gets weaker and wiser the doctors has gotten to the place and science has gotten to the place they makes all these other medicines to take the place of those old Indian remedies. You don't have to have so much of it now. Befo it wasn't to be bought.

I'll tell you another remedy they had for he'pin the baby for teethin. They would take a piece of fat hog meat and a real fat piece of splinter. Stick that piece of fat on there and hold it over a saucer and let the turpentine, the resin from that fat piece of splinter, and the fat meat drop down together. They would take that and rub the baby's gums with it where it was teethin. I can remember that. Make a salve to rub his gums. I can remember my mother doin this. Those lil wood chips—put em right in the bag and tie em round the baby's neck for teethin. I don't fault em for that cause that's all anybody knew in those days. You have to live and learn. They did too. They had a long ways to come. That was medication through faith healin. Whatever they'd use God led it through His knowledge and it worked because they didn't have nothin else to work with.

I never will fo'get. In the swamp part of our farm the weeds they grows up like this. All kinda weeds so we can cut it and make hay for the cows in wintertime. My sister Betty—they always cuttin and they could sharpen those hoes as sharp as they could be and they'd go one right behind the other cuttin. Oh—that was a beautiful life. Somebody lef their hoe under that dried grass and my sister Betty stepped on it and cut the bottom of her heel, you know, the thick part. Almost to the bone all the way across. All the way across. In these days you would got a lockjaw seal and was dead befo tomorrow if you hadn't go gotten and taken a shot. It was laid open like that.

Mother taken her to the house and prayed and with the he'p of God she went out and got—there was a big can of axle grease that Daddy used to grease the wheels of his wagon with so they could roll easy. She filled that whole place—cleaned the blood and the sand out and she filled that place full of axle grease. About an hour later he come—it used to be a man goin around sellin different medicines or grease or salves and such as. Here he come along with the same grease. Looked exactly like axle grease other than probably have a lil medicine care in it. She bought that. She kep that place full of axle grease and that salve too and it healed up. Betty was fat and was chubby and when she stepped on that hoe it laid that place open almost an inch deep wide open. Hadn't seen any doctor. Mother kep it up. She kep it clean. She didn't let no sand get in it and prayed and it healed. It healed. She woulda needed three tetanus shots in these days. I'm talkin bout what I looked at with these eyes. What happen when I know. A miracle is the word. Just laid open.

She cleaned it and bandaged it up and she wouldn't let her walk in the sand. She bandaged it up with different clean rags and kep a sock on it. She made her stay off the sand for a couple a days or mo days. Several days I would say and when she started hoppin around on it she kep it secure from grit. So no grit or nothin couldn't heal up in it and she would dress it ever day. She knew she wasn't go'n get no doctor. She knew wasn't one comin out. To go to catch him in his office is every now and then you can catch him. God takes care of that person that don't know and doin the best he can. He gets in there and work. A lot a people don't know why it works but I thank God I do know why it works. Cause the Lord aim for it to work. They're doin the best they can. But was the Lord healin all the time.

That was the worst I ever seen her. When she stepped on that sharp hoe, it just laid this heel up under there. Mother washed it. She prayed. She got all the sand out of it and then she went out there and got this axle grease and she just leveled it off with axle grease. Late that evenin here come this man with a big box of almost the same stuff as that axle grease. It was black just like that axle grease but it had a different smell to it. You could smell somethin else in it and it worked.

I didn't use as much of those old remedies. I didn't use it cause really along about my time they was plenty of medicine that you could go buy. Vicks salve for fever and for colds but I always have said it's made out the same stuff that lil weed is. See all a that start comin in that you could go to the drugsto or you could go to the sto and buy it durin my time. So I didn't have to deal with those home cures but I've heard of it so much so until I know they used it in those days. I'm glad I wasn't here to have to in those times. With all a that science I didn't have to come in contact with so much a that other stuff. But you know it took me a long time. Women in those days they just beginnin to get away from it. Especially our black girls. They want to continue to do like what mother said and grandmother said. It hadn't been too long they've gotten away from all that. I can see why. I don't blame em. That's what their old grandparents brought em up on. It hadn't been too long they got away from that.

Those old midwives in those days was black v
doin it for a job but doin it as a person knowin thei
for it. They were doin the very best they could
wouldn't criticize em so much because they were doin the best
they could and doin a job well done as fur as their knowledge
would lead em. I don't call that ignorant. That's tryin to help
doin the best they can with the knowledge they have. Tryin to
help where the doctors didn't come around to help or didn't
make preparations to help. The person with all the knowledge
and all the sense didn't come around and didn't make no effort
and didn't do nothin. I don't say she wasn't filthy. I don't say
she wasn't uncompetent. Those old Negroes in those days
needed trainin.

What I'm talkin about is the death of so many mothers and
babies in those times, and the midwife was blamed. That was
not the midwife. That was the lackin of prenatal care. No
vitamins, no calciums. No prenatal care whatsoever. It was not
havin proper food. Not havin enough calcium for her and baby.
Probably not havin any for either one of em cause usually when
the baby is to be bo'n he get all the calcium from mother. If
mother ain't got enough for both of em that baby get every drop
she got. If you ain't got enough for both of you shame on you.
A lot a times in those days they didn't have enough for the baby
much less for both of em cause they hadn't had prenatal care. It
wasn't because a the midwives. They had to lay the situation
on somebody and so they laid it on the midwives. Those
midwives—their fingers don't have to touch the birth canal. If
the filth was there it was because the bed and the clothe;
quite sanitary. If they get that fever it don't have

directly from the fingers. Childbirth fever is mostly a natural thing that will happen to you. The causes I don't know. If it comes from the midwives, there wouldn't be hardly all these babies that these black people and these po white people had that lived in the country and on the farms.

Mostly older Negro womens and then some of the white did make their pipe and smoke a co'ncob pipe. I'm not go'n say that they didn't do it cause they did smoke pipes at that time. I've seen the snuff dippin and the tobacco chewin. I don't say with midwives. With women. A lot of em did it in those days. In those olden days like that most women they dip their snuff. Most of em dip snuff or they chew tobacco. They would make their pipe outa co'ncob. I remember my Aunt Mandy and even my daddy—my mother didn't smoke a pipe—but I remember them makin their nice pipes outa co'ncob. They hollow the center of it out and lef the bottom part where it didn't go around through and over the top part and get em a piece a cane and make a hole through it and bore a hole in the co'ncob and stick it in there and fill it up full a their homemade tobacco and smoked it. My father grew all his tobacco. He sold some of it. Didn't have a whole lot. You just work yo tobacco where you plant it it just multiplies. It didn't take a whole lot to last him from one season to the other. I would say they was greasy nasty filthy uncompetent women cause they hadn't been taught.

I've always from a lil girl wanted to be a nurse. Bein a nurse started young when I was a child, nursin my lil sick baby doll. We made our dolls. There's a weed and when you pull up this weed it's got a lot a roots to it, long like that. We would lay it

68

out in the sun and let it dry and that was the hair and we would tie this lil string around the green part of it and then there was the lil head and the hair. We would keep them lil things—just gobs of em—and work with em as our lil doll. Mother would give us a button, a small button, that has come off. She would give us anything that we could dot here for the lil eyes and the lil mouth and we got a thrill outa that just like they do the dolls now. We made a lot of em outa rags. We had so many old homemade dolls and their hair was—we'd taken old rags and just slitted it up and make it fine to play with. There wasn't no other dolls to be bought then. The doll I had was always sick. That deal with me all the time. I was always a nurse for my baby cause my baby was always sick. That was when it began when I was that young. The Lord deal to me in visions to be a person to he'p somebody. When I was young I had that vision over and over and over again. I'd get those visions that my doll was sick and I was the nurse with the doll. As I grew there was people that I was havin visions about that I needed to help. Just anybody. I was he'pin somebody not knowin exactly who it was. Sometime it would be a person that I know. And then again it just be he'pin somebody. It was my doll when I's very little.

When my mother used to visit—I never will fo'get. When I's quite a lil girl my mother was visitin, she was takin care of an old Mr. Warren Robinson and his sister. White. Brother and sister that never had been married, lived together in an old homestead. Lived in a big red house. Their parents who naturally I didn't know left em in this great big nice two-story house—that brother and sister. It was a nice place. Real nice place. My mother would go there to take care Miss Cynthia—that was her name—taken sick first. My mother went to see her day and night. She stayed there a many night all night. I slep on the flo on a lil quilt and my mother would sit by that lady all night when she was sick. And then Mother would want to go home. Not fur from home. Not too fur from home. She would want me to stay there. She would say, "Onnie, I want you to sit here and fan Miss Cynthia." No fans, no nothin. Hot. And I would sit there for hours and fan that lady. I remember that just as well and fan her till Mother go and come back. Little girl—eleven or twelve years old. And my mother would bathe her and fix her up and feed her and I watched Mother tendin to her.

Several people like that. And she would tell me that she wanted me to fan em or she would tell me "I want you to hold em" when she turn em. She said hold her shoulders—lil girl—while I turn the body for her. She was just that sick. Hardly no hospitals or nothin then. Now and then you could get a doctor. So I would watch Mother and my heart went out to he'p somebody right then and there. A lil girl, I could go to bed and go to sleep seein myself fannin Miss Cynthia or seein myself fannin Miss Rose Harris. Now those are the people that I went with Mother to see. Mother would carry me always. Privilege for me from the rest of em. Cause I was eager to he'p. I wanted to he'p. And that's what we did. That was another one of the guidance from God, who guided my mind each and every day that my mother taught me. Use whatcha got. Use whatcha got. And I used it to the best of my knowledge and God give me or my mother would he'p me get through with that. If I hadn't had guidance from God I woulda just gotten preserve a myself. I ask God to guide me and Mother asked God to guide me too and direct me in the right path and the right way to go beyond myself to get along with ever'body. "Now, Onnie," she said. "Love ever'body." Love, share, and care and that's what I do right now and I done that from a lil girl all my life.

Miss Cynthia told my mother that she was go'n die—she was not go'n live. Said, "When I die I don't want nobody but you to bathe me." At that time you didn't send em to the undertaker parlor. You dressed em the next day or the same day and got em ready for bur'al. She said, "When I die I want nobody to come in here and to see you bathin me. I want you to bathe me yo'self just like you done all the time." About three days befo she died she told Mother what slip to get her, what dress to put on her, and Mother had all a that layin out. And Mother carried it out just like she told her. And dressed her. Mother washed and dressed all over the county. When she dressed her, naturally, they brought the casket to the house in those days. Remember I told you my daddy made their caskets. And they brought the casket in after Mother dressed her and got her all fixed up. No makeup in those days but they would get a lil powder and try to smooth the face up a lil bit. There were other white ladies standin around watchin. Miss Cynthia had friends, you know, that wanted to do or probably would do, but they wasn't go'n go that far naturally. Some of her friends, I guess they felt like they shoulda been there. I think she told some of em that "when I die, Tinny go'n take care a me." Then the men brought the casket in and then the men put her in the casket. But getting her dressed and ready Mother did.

71

And she did the same thing for Miss Cynthia's brother fo or five years later he died. And I myself then was beginnin to get to be around fo'teen or fifteen years old or mo. Bathed him a many a time. I tell you, Mother sent me down there one mornin to scramble him some eggs, give him some jelly and bread. I don't know what the reason that she couldn't go but I goes down to feed him and to milk the cow for him. And he had fallen outa the bed he was just that sick. And he had feces all over. All over the bed and all over him. I had a time but I want you to know that lil girl worked with it until she got it all off. And put on him mo clothes myself. That's a white man. I did that. And that's my idea of wantin to he'p somebody. That's the way we had to do durin that time cause there was no hospitals worth anything that people were able to go to. Wasn't hardly any to go to. We just used our wisdom and knowledge as God give us how to take care of one another in those days until we died. Just took care of one another. No hospitals then and few doctors.

They paid my mother such as it was. Such as it was they had ever'thing. They had plenty in which we had plenty of too. Plenty of fruit. Mother could go down there when she was cannin fruit and she would churn and she would have mo butter and mo milk to carry home. And we wheeled the stuff to carry home and feed our ho'se with from the Robinsons from milkin their cows.

When I was about I imagine fifteen, I was a maid in a white home. That was Mrs. Addison. Mother did her clothes along with all them others. They owned the grocery sto in that great big sawmill quarter in Sweet Water. She asked Mother to let me come down to he'p her. She had a lil boy named Joseph Addison. Mostly she wanted Mother to let me come and entertain that child. I would go mornin's down to Mrs. Addison. She's a big stout woman. Very big and fat. Friendly as she could be but you know how big peoples are. They're lazy. They ain't lazy but they just hate to move about. Those kinda people didn't get around much cause they're so heavy. When she knew that I knew about cleanin house and cookin she put me to sweepin and dustin and started me cookin vegetables and bread and start fryin chicken. See Mother would teach us ever'thing from here on up. So then from there I just started doin ever'thing there was to be done. Ever'thing that I could get done. I did ever'thing just like a grown-up woman. She didn't pay me well in that time. That was at least fifty-five years ago. I cain't remember what I was getting cause what lil it was I carried it straight home to Mother. It wasn't that much. I was in the bedroom when she had her next baby. That was Dr. Jones in Sweet Water. He never said anything to me. There was quite a big prejudice about him. He just didn't have too much to say, just didn't pay too much attention to me. I nursed her and baby at my age of sixteen. She made me nurse the baby and bathe the baby. I cared for em and then did the cookin.

Not only that, my mother would send me down to tend and bathe my sisters' and brothers' babies. I got my good experience by bathin. That's where I got my start. That gave me experience in my early days—teenage. That just grew at me. That's what I want to be. It really did. It just expand in me that that's the job I want and I tried so hard. Mother told me, she said, "You've got to study to be gettin it. You've got to study to do nurse work."

As I said, my mother had taken sick and died and that just taken schoolin away from me cause I didn't have nobody to push me. She was gone and there was Daddy with all the rest of them chil'rens and that just killed my sense. When Mother died that just took all the spirit from me for school. It probably wouldn't've did like that but she told us what to do on her deathbed. "Try to take care of one another. Try to take care of your daddy." I was just so full I didn't see myself bein away and tryin to do what she said but I still had in my mind that I was gonna be a nurse.

I never will fo'get it was Sunday night durin a meetin that my mother and daddy have always done. If we didn't get to go back to church we would have prayer meetin's on Sunday night and we would stay at home like I told you. So we were havin prayer meetin and my sisters and brothers that lived on the place, they would come all like family and we would have prayer meetin. A couple of neighbors. My mother had a stroke and was prayin the last prayer durin service that night at home. I could just hear her voice the way she prays right now. She kep gettin lower and lower and lower the voice. I stood up and I looked around and Daddy sittin over there and he done stood up cause we would bow and get on our knees right by the chair where she was sittin. Never did hear when she ended her prayer but she stood up and Dad said, "What's the matter, hon?" That's what he called her all the time. By that time we'd all gotten around her and she says nothin. You could hear her mumble and you understood what she was sayin. "Nothin the matter with me." She said, "Get me a drink a water." When she said that she didn't say nothin else. We couldn't understand anything else she said for three weeks. Daddy went to get water and a towel and go get Dr. Jones. Daddy run up to Sweet Water to the lil town and got Dr. Jones and he didn't come. Just didn't get outa bed. That's just the way it was in the country and with the colored people.

She lived seven weeks. She came back long enough to tell us ever'thing she wanted us to do. She told us to take care of one another and when one of us gotten sick don't one wait on the other to he'p. "All of you go see bout that one that needs you and take care of yo daddy. Ada—that was the oldest sister who was old enough for my mother herself—she said "I want you to see about Daddy's clothes. Keep em washed and ironed in the place where I would." She said, "I want you to do that. Nettie, I want you to do this and I want you to do that. Onnie, I want you to go see about the clothes. When Daddy buy all his gingham I want you to still make their clothes to work in." She stayed with us but still sick. She said, "I'm tellin all a you this now while I can." She said, "You remember when I had my last baby?"—which was J.B. "I remember when he was born." She says, "I taken real sick when he was born. I asked Him to spare me till my baby get up big enough to take care a hisself." She said, "Now he's thirteen or fo'teen years old and I'm not go'n ask God to save me. I'm ready to go cause He ready for me to go." She died that Thursday night at seven o'clock.

I was around eighteen years old when my mother died. I was just gettin ready for high school. When Mother died it discouraged me from my schoolin. And I wasn't so well either. At that time I wasn't so well. I was just a lil puny girl. I stayed home and tend to ever'thing while the rest of em worked in the fields. When I lost her I was at a loss. I didn't have nobody to go ask. I always ask what I don't know. I didn't try to go on and did it myself unless I knew what I was doin. I was lost. That's the very reason I didn't go on to school. I was lost. I couldn't find myself. I really was. I found myself later. But went I shoulda went on to school and further my education and further in what I wanted to do I couldn't do it. I couldn't read. I couldn't study. I could sit down and get a book and go to readin. I'd start cryin late at night for a long time.

Vocation

I lef Sweet Water, I was about twenty-one when I got married for the first time. I married a brother to my sister Evie's husband. We married brothers. I thought Louise, my sister Evie Louise, had a fairly good husband. I thought it was just wonderful that I was goin to marry his brother. So it went along like that. Come to find out that I married nothin. He wanted every woman he saw, every one. I was married about a month. Then I was pregnant. Then he in turns walks off from me with the baby with another woman and that was it. I gave him a full chance for about three years. For that long. I didn't want to happen what did happen cause that ain't what I married him for. I wanted to make it if you can and I tried. That's all he ever done was to chase women. Just not come home. When he'd come home it was a fight and a pull. In that time people didn't hardly have nothin to eat. I got married durin the Depression. You know no money. Fifty-two years ago, fifty-one years ago wasn't a nickel. We was livin in Magnolia, Alabama. My husband was doin nothin. He worked quite a lil on the railroad track. The mens have to keep the tracks up and goin all the time. He was just workin wherever he could. He didn't have no regular job. In the country in those days, mighty few people work. They work when they can and where they can.

When I was livin in Magnolia, Magnolia was in its good blooms. It was an up town and on one a the railroads. Was built on a railroad since they built that Frisco Railroad through there. Now that's what you call downtown. It was a depot there, a

77

post office there, a grocery sto there, a lil motel-hotel there cause right there is where the mens that come in on those trains that work trains would spend the night. The ones out from Pensacola would spend the night there and they'd go back to Pensacola and these from Meridian would go back up in Mississippi. On out fu'ther is what you call old Magnolia. They be outstandin people—white people—lived in there. Old Magnolia is where Dr. Guilliard lived. Some of em had the big houses. Some of em was wealthy as wealthy was in those days. The black people lived around the country in the field. Farms. That's a lil country place. That was a lil depot town on the railroad where that railroad went through there. That was a lil depot town.

My sister-in-law was workin at the hotel as they would call it. Cook there. Then there would be depot agents' wives around that these men that was workin on the train. They spent the night there and went back the next mornin. The ones from Memphis and back up in Mississippi and outa Pensacola would then turn to have their clothes washed then. A lot of us did washin of their clothes, the men's clothes. They would take a bath naturally to go to bed and they'd change their clothes. They had a change here and a change where they come from home. I did some a that. And I also worked with several ladies, white ladies around that area.

I was workin with one lady, she was originally from Meridian, Mississippi, and her husband was workin the railroad there. They was livin upstairs at the Frisco Railroad Depot. He was a depot agent and his office was downstairs. I was workin for her when Dr. Guilliard would make his visits there to see her and he would have conversations with me about deliveries and babies. I was there with him when the baby was born. Dr. Guilliard told me, says, "Well," he says, "you got to he'p me. You got to be my nurse today." I said, "Well, good," and I got scrubbed up and ready. I was then about twenty-one or twenty-two. Twenty-one or twenty-two. I got Dr. Guilliard's water ready. At that time there wasn't runnin water and I got his water ready. Shoved on his gloves. When he asked for this that was there. This and that was there. I had it all ready for him. And then when she got ready to have it Dr. Guilliard took a sheet and he carried it around that iron. I never will fo'get. She was in a iron bed and he put that sheet around that bed and he tied two square knots in there. She took them knots and she pulled when she had those hard contractions.

I was up at her head and I was talkin to her while she was havin contractions. I said, "Miss Stephanie, you're doin fine. Keep yo mind on what you're doin and I believe that would keep you from screamin." I kep tellin her to keep an eye on what you're doin and what's happenin. That's the impo'tant thing. And sooner or later it'll be over with. Not this minute but sooner or later. That contraction will ease. Not knowin what the doctor was thinkin but I kep on with that all the time all the way through. He could hear me when I said, "Don't push too hard." And she'd come again. And I'd say, "Use just a lil bit mo pressure." And I'd say, "Don't cut em too sharp. Hold a lil longer. Not too hard but just a lil longer." I coached her right on through that along with him. And I hadn't had my own baby yet. I was just coachin her what to do and what not to do. I didn't give him a chance to do it. That's how come he was givin me the eye. I know he was wonderin "Where is that comin from?" And that's when he asked me wanted to know where'd I get trainin.

I can remember Dr. Guilliarn showed me how to tie a cord. They didn't have clamps then at all. They used a sterile tie but now they have clamps. He wanted me to come and watch him tie the cord, cut the cord. Then when he did that he'd do precisely like we do now. Lay the baby on mother's breast while he was examinin her and getting her all ready. Then I had to clean the baby and straighten up the mother. He was surprised at the way I taken care of the baby and mother. As soon as he finished he sit down and have a long conversation with me and he said, "You would make a good midwife. Not only make a good midwife. I think you'll make a good doctor." I hadn't had any experience. It was right in there and it was time for it to start comin out. And it did. Dr. Guilliard got up my courage that I should be a good midwife. That was a goal I made to myself right then and there. I started makin that goal as a midwife. I knew I couldn't get it unless I kep workin towards it. It was not comin to me. I had to go get it. I never will fo'get that boy was named Carl.

When I got my baby, got pregnant, they told me you'll have that baby within nine months. Nobody had told me nothin else. I got me a calendar and I sit down and I said I supposed to menstruate right here and I didn't. I supposed to menstruate right here the next month and there the next month. I counted it up to the very day my baby was born. On the very day that I had already counted up without anybody tellin me anything and it was born on the twenty-ninth. I said, "I'm go'n eat up all that Christmas stuff. I'm go'n eat it and then I'm go'n have my baby." I had it on the twenty-ninth and I knew from the second month when I was pregnant. Nobody had told me nothin about childbirth. Nobody to really talk to and Mother was dead. Nobody to tell you exactly how it is. I didn't know nothin about it. Nobody to tell me nothin about it. Nobody hadn't told me how to take care of myself.

I was such a lil thin girl my daddy wanted me back with my older sisters. I went down maybe a couple a weeks befo gettin in labor to my brother Sid's house and had my one child in his house just below the old homestead. When I got in labor my sister-in-law had to go over across the field where my daddy was workin to get him to go get the midwife. So he went by and got the car and went over to Thelma's. She did a good job considerin what midwives knew in those days. In those days they made women bear to their contractions too long. They didn't know no better. They start em pushin almost as soon as they got in labor.

I got in labor early that mornin about sunup. I was lyin there in the bed and I could hear my sister-in-law in the kitchen gettin my brother off to work. I felt somethin funny. I had never felt that befo. I laid there for about fo'ty-five minutes or an hour. There was another one which lasted a lil bit longer. I said, "I better get up," and went across towards my other sister-in-law that lived right across the branch up there. I started over there and I got down to the branch and one super one. I had to go to my knees. I said, "I better go back." So I went back to the house and then that's when I told my sister-in-law and she was nervous as a cricket. Had been married about eight years and hadn't had any chil'ren and she got upset and she ran across the field over there to tell Dad to come. At that time I hadn't had another one. And he came on and another one come and Dad run in. He was worried about me. He said, "I wished plenty times I had died befo yo mother did cause I didn't know what to do with all these girls." He asked me how I was feelin. I said, "Dad, I feel all right but." Out he went to get the midwife. She musta came in about ten-thirty or eleven o'clock and the baby was bo'n about six.

She stayed the whole time. I have stayed twenty-fo hours. She wasn't there but about six, seven hours. Now that's pretty good bein yo first baby. To make me comfortable she had me in bed. Contractions got so severe. In those days they let you have yo baby on the flo anyway. They got a crib and padded that crib and you had yo baby there if you wanted to or when the baby got ready to be bo'n they let you get on yo knees outside of the bed or on a chair sittin by the bed and you had yo baby there. You had a better bearin the last minute contractions. You could cope with em better. I had mine on my knees. I had been up walkin around and in bed and outa bed but when it come time for it to come through the birth canal I got on my knees. That's what she said would suit you better. You better get down on yo knees.

I don't think Elmo had any chil'ren by other women. Befo I had had the child from him they said, "Well one thing about it," ever'body said, "Big Buddy wasn't able to get no child and didn't have no chil'ren." I can remember they all called him Big Buddy, the family did. Wasn't go'n have this. But he sure was lucky to get that one. That's the only child that he had. A lot a women's would just lay a baby on a man. He's the daddy of this So-and-So's child. He's the daddy of So-and-So's child. They said he hadn't had any baby laid on him.

I had that baby musta been eleven months after we got married. That baby was born eleven months after we was married. And then I had a miscarriage after the first baby. I had my only child. Elmo wasn't a father at all. He wasn't home long enough. He didn't hate him. He didn't mistreat him and didn't bruise him or nothin like that. He wasn't home long enough to show the love that a father would show for his child. Daddy never talked too much against him but he would say how sorry he was and this, that, and the other. Elmo went down and beat my daddy outa some money once. Said that I needed it and sent for it when we were livin in Magnolia and I didn't even know it. Not at all.

I can remember the time there was a lady. I lived in a lil house in the bottom near the railroad track in Magnolia. There was a lady that lived on the hill and she wanted some washin done. I put my baby to sleep in that lil house and I went up there. I guess I was takin chances and prayin that my child was still sleepin while I's workin. Washed, boiled the clothes. Rinsed em and hung em out on the line to get some milk and some meal and a couple a eggs. Saved those eggs for my baby's breakfast and she gave me a can a beans. I come home and open those beans. Had that milk and bread and those beans for supper that night and saved the two eggs to scramble with some rice for my baby's breakfast that mornin. We got along. Me and the baby. There was enough to make it there all the time. Enough to survive without the sufferin. You know what? Had I not stuck with the salvation of the Lord and kep him in front to guide, I wouldn't have rose above that. What I cain't do for myself and I don't see my way out I depends on the Lord and it opens up. That's how I survived. That's how I didn't pay no attention to it bein as hard as it was.

I come in contact with several other midwives up in Magnolia. Now this midwife, I was with her on several occasions with my in-laws. She worked precisely just like an old country midwife would. Wore them long aprons. My husband's sister's chil'ren, my sister-in-law, she had fo girls that had babies. I went with the midwife on all those deliveries. She did a good job considerin that's the best a their knowledge in those days. I didn't like it. I was so glad I didn't come on durin that time. They make peoples start pressin down to their contractions as soon as they start. Start pushin right off. They did that. So you know what? It was hard on the patient. If you start a patient pushin down too early you'll prolong the labor instead a speedin it up. That's what they thought it did. They never did know any better. I would always did that different. I'm glad I wasn't a midwife durin that time.

I would say they taught me lil pieces here and there. I was always anxious to learn and get started on whatever it take to be a good midwife. It just come to me from them. When they was teachin me this in my mind I was addin a lit bit mo to it. I could do it like them. That's exactly the way I come about mine. I was watchin and takin in what they was sayin but I always see'd it a lil different that you could do or you could add to it. And that's the way I progressed. Mo and mo like that. That's how come I say God give it to me. The Bo'd a Health didn't give it to me. Readin books didn't give it to me. I progressed that outa my own mind. My own mind. Thinkin and listenin and knowledge that God give me.

I moved from Magnolia to Mobile. That musta been in 'thirty-three, 'thirty-fo. At that time my baby was about three years old. My husband got a job workin with cross-ties on the railroad tracks. Frisco and L&N. They moved here to Mobile and that's when I came to Mobile.

When we first got to Mobile I started workin for Mrs. Wilson down on Murray Street. I started workin at 101 Murray Street and I was makin only a dollar and a half for five days. For five days. I went for a dollar and a half a week as a maid. I knew that you wouldn't want to believe, but that's the way it was. Mrs. Wilson was my husband's boss man's wife. That's how I got that job. That's how I got that. Elmo was with them boys loadin those ties on the railroad from one place to the other all the way up and down the Frisco Railroad and the L&N Railroad. Where the trucks was haulin them ties they would load em on the boxcar on the truck. That's what he was doin.

He had a good job when other mens around here wasn't workin or makin nothin. When they could've brought home fifty and sixty dollars a week, that's two hundred dollars these days. That was big money. He didn't make it home with not a dime. They knew he didn't come home. They knew he didn't bring me much and when they asked me I didn't hide it. Mr. Wilson, he would ask me, tell me say, "Well I know Elmo made it home with some good money this week," but I would tell him how it really stood with me.

Then finally Elmo up and lef with this other lady. I did the best I could and went to get my divo'ce. Durin askin questions—I had a lady for a lawyer. She asked questions and asked questions. I told her right then that I come to find out Elmo was already married and never had been divo'ced from that yet. She said, "Well you got no divo'ce to get. You wasn't married in the first place." I had done found out from relatives and friends up there as I met people in Magnolia. They told me. His own relatives told me that he had done been married befo. I was so upset and worried I didn't even ask questions about that until time come to get my divo'ce. That just killed me as fur as mens concerned for a long time. But I never stopped doin somethin to increase my life, my feelin. I kep church work goin all the time to keep me from worryin about the situation that was happenin right through then.

I was a maid for Dr. Mears. They had ads in the paper. It's a big white house, sits way back, long tall columns. I lived out there on the place. My lil place was in the back. I had a bedroom and a bath. We eat all our meals in the kitchen. I did everything there was to be done. The hours wasn't limited. The hours was not limited. And that was durin the time that they worked you, honey, especially if you was livin on the place. That was durin when you was workin for about a dollar and a half a week. And that wasn't bad durin that time at all. Not at all and I accepted it with a smile. I thought that's the way we should live. That's the way we were. It has changed so much for the better and I thank God for it. But at the time I didn't let that part worry me. That didn't go through my mind. We just lived. We lived and made ourselves happy about it. The way Dr. Mears and them lived—I felt like that's what they supposed to be like. That's what they were. White folks. That's what white folks supposed to be like. That's the way it meant to be at that time. If it didn't meant to be like that it woulda been different. But I didn't let that go through my mind. I lived as a human bein and I treated you as a human bein and lef the rest up to God.

Mrs. Mears was young when I started workin for her. And I was young too. We was both about the same age. I believe we was in our late twenties. We was. We was in our late twenties. And I was there befo she was pregnant with her first baby. And then I was there when she had all three chil'rens so I raised those chil'rens like they was my own and they love me like that right today. I never will fo'get. Dr. Mears and Mrs. Mears went to Europe one year and I had to go to the hospital. The minute those chil'rens knew I was there, it was either one or the other one was there every day to see about me. Now that's the way they feel about me. They know that's the way I feel about them.

I work for now, Mrs. Simpson, said she don't know
could like Southerners because of the situation and the
way we was treated. Mrs. Simpson wouldn't want you to call
her a Southerner. No, she's not a Southerner. She wouldn't
want to be called that cause she thinks they are—she thinks
they are dumb, stupid and awful. She thinks these Southerners
is trash. That's what she called em. She talks about the
Southerners this and the Southerners that. Cain't get em to do
this. Cain't get em to do nothin but sit down. They ain't good
for breathin that old hot air which ain't nothin. Co'se I wasn't
in the category she was talkin about although I was a
Southerner. So that include me too in a way.

When I told Dr. Mears I wanted to be a midwife he thought
it was a wonderful job. He has been a wonderful, wonderful
person to me. We are in the same category, that we love to he'p
somebody. He has always helped me with his ideas and
thoughts. I don't think there's nothin that I would ever need
that I wouldn't get if I need it from Dr. Mears or Mrs. Mears. I
don't think Mrs. Mears thought it was a wonderful job cause
she thought I was gonna move off the place. She liked me so
well as a maid. I believe she thought I was gonna move off but
I was there.

That was when I started goin to class. I got into it with a
couple of midwives that was here and they wanted me to come
to the Bo'd a Health and take a midwife co'se at the Bo'd a
Health. So I did that. There was a Mrs. Tyler was my instructor.
She was the instructor there. It was just about a year befo they
issued me my permit because I had good standin from all

beginnin. Befo movin to Mobile I was with several an..
midwives plus two doctors. That helped em to give me my
permit. I got a permit quicker than any midwife that was in
Mobile. I had experience. I brought in all a the deliveries I had
had befo I come to Mobile. I was licensed after that. I got my
first permit in 1949.

Just a few months befo I got my first permit, I went around
with a midwife who done already got her permit for three
deliveries. Apprentice. I went with one midwife that she
delivered twins. She delivered twins. The first baby were born.
She tried and she couldn't get it to breathe or nothin so she laid
it down. When she laid it down I picked it up and I started
workin with it. She said, "Oh, Mamie, you got another baby
comin." She said, "You got twins." Well she delivered that baby
and cleaned it up and dressed it and she got cleaned up the
mother and dressed her. I was still workin with that other one.
"Lay it down, Onnie, it's dead. I worked with that baby for
fo'ty-five minutes. I got a heartbeat and I got breathin. That's
when I started dependin on my own experience. I pitched out
on what God told me to do then. I forgot about books and other
people. Well I worked on that lil child and I worked on it.

At that time they didn't have Pampers—they had these
bird-eye diapers. I grabbed me a clean bird-eye diaper and I
blowed in his mouth with mouth-to-mouth resuscitation. I
hadn't been taught that. Didn't know anything about it but
that's what I did. I did that and I picked it up with my hands
under its lil ribs on its lil back and I feel that lil faint heart beatin
about thirty minutes later. When I did that I filled it full of wind

again then I would take my hand and take the lil stomach and pump it out like breathin. That lil heart just come getting a lil bit stronger and stronger. So I did that about fo times, filled it full of wind with my mouth on its mouth. So finally it kep that and I'd take my hand off its lil stomach where I was pumpin and then it kep goin. I'd feel that breath gettin stronger and stronger and stronger. Fo'ty-five minutes I worked on that baby and I had never delivered a baby befo. I had never done mouth-to-mouth resuscitation.

You know why I did that? I asked God to he'p me to bring that baby to life if life was in it and He gave me power to do it. I learned then who to depend on from that. That's what I did and that boy's married and got a house full a chil'rens. Sho is. That was a black boy. The other midwife kep tellin me lay it down, it's gone. Lay it down. She couldn't believe it. She said, "I never woulda known." I examined that child. I felt that lil heart. He just fit in the palm a my hand. I caught him right up under the ribs with this hand and this thumb was on where the lil heart was and that's where I felt that lil heartbeat every once in a while. Very, very faint. The next time I felt it breathin in and pumpin out. No ma'am I hadn't been taught how to do that.

I progressed that outa my mind. My own mind. There was a higher power and God give me wisdom. Motherwit, common sense. Wisdom come from on high. You got it and you cain't explain how you got it yo'self. It's motherwit. I cain't tell you exactly how I got it or I cain't tell exactly how Mother did it. Listenin at the classes I would say helped a lot. It grew within my mind what to expect and what to think about. All at the same time God was talkin to me cause I was so interested. You know if you love yo job you can do anything. I would say the classes taught me how to make the pads. The classes taught me beginning a scrubbin up my hands. The classes taught me how to tie the cord. The classes taught me how to put the silver nitrate in the babies' eyes. The classes taught me how to make my bag, how to pack my bag, and all a that. What goes in the bag. But so many things that I have run into the classes did not teach me. The classes did not teach me so many things. I can only put it this way and I can be for sho that I'm right. Two-thirds of what I know about deliverin, carin for mother and baby, what to expect, what was happenin and was goin on, I didn't get from the class. God give it to me. So many things I got from my own plain motherwit.

That first baby is a lesson to let you know. This first baby that I delivered I knew the mother well. Not directly but indirectly we were friends. She told me, "I'm gonna let you deliver my baby." I said, "Really." She said, "Yeah." I said, "Good for you." I really didn't go to the trouble to tell her that that was my first baby. It was breeched, my very first baby. And that didn't scare me at all. I've never had a job that scared me. I do believe and I do know there is a higher power. And He certainly will direct yo path if you let Him. If you will trust Him, if you will serve Him, He will direct yo path. He's not gonna let you make a mistake as long as you're workin in His name.

Now they tell us not to deliver a breech baby. The way you know the baby is breech even befo the lil butt shows up good that cain't hardly tell the buttocks from the head—you get this black feces first. You don't guide the breech baby out cause as soon as the lil butt comes, the lil hands is like this, you see, and the lil feets is up like this and the butt is comin first. I o'dered the doctor in time enough. It was a Dr. Muskat and I called him. He says, "Well how is things comin?" I said, "Well she had a good labor but the lil buttocks comin first." He said, "Well, I reckon I better get up and get my clothes on and get on out there to you." But he didn't have to come. The Lord said, "Now you don't need Dr. Muskat. You can handle this," and there was the baby. About three or fo minutes later I had delivered that breech birth and that was my first baby and I did it all by myself. Beautiful. Befo that doctor could get outa bed at two o'clock in the morning, befo he could get outa bed and get dressed, I had the privilege of callin him back and tellin him everything was fine and the baby was here and mother and baby was fine. That was about two o'clock in the morning and he said, "Thank you, Onnie, I'll get my clothes back off and go to bed," and that's what he did.

Durin the first ten years of my career as a midwife, it was mainly black families I delivered for. Those black families I was deliverin for, they was po. Especially durin the first times they was po. Hardly nothin but po in those days. It was po times. It really was—no jobs. When I first started to work the houses of the black neighborhoods, some of the houses was about the same as the houses in Sweet Water. They was livin in houses that—mostly as they used to call em—shotgun houses. There was probably two bedrooms and a lil kitchen. That's it for huge families. No livin room. No bathroom. No nothin. Just two bedrooms and a kitchen for most of em. Maybe a po'ch. Most of em in those times in the bedrooms they would squeeze in two beds to the room. It would always mostly have two beds to a room and a cot for em to sleep. For all of em. Three or fo sleep with the parents. Five or six with the parents. Especially with the general run of em. The kids learned about the facts a life in the bed with the parents. It was like that. It's just like animals. That went on all the time in those days.

Most of em had wood heaters to heat their house. Them old wood heaters and old-timey lil fireplaces. There wasn't any gas hardly around in those places. These lil old wood heaters for cold winter days and these lil bitty fireplaces. Their kitchen would have a lil woodstove and a lil table. Mostly they didn't have chairs or nothin to sit down in. They stood up or sit on the flo to eat their food. No electricity. They had kerosene lamps. I delivered many a baby by kerosene lamps. No runnin water. You had to sterile yo water—boil it. You got it outside and brought it inside. They had an outside toilet. They used those lil aluminum washtubs, lil tin tubs as they call em. They'd carry it in the kitchen and heat you some water. Most places they would have to pump their water outside. As my parents have said, we have come a long, long ways. I really didn't pay too much attention to it bein hard. I take it as it comes. Just what need to be done. What they got I can use it. I think that's a pretty good way to be.

Mostly the general run of em they kep their place clean although it was a small place and it was the best they could do. They kep it presentable. There are plenty people would clean up their house period if they didn't have nothin but to pull off this dress and wash it and let it dry and put it back on. They'd clean it. And then there's some of em would just wear that old floppy dress until it would just fall off em. Get so slick and greasy.

In those days I had to go out and have a meetin with em befo I delivered their baby. When they engage you that they wanted you to deliver their baby, you in turns would have to make from two to three trips to visit that mother to outline things, to see how the situation was goin on, and to he'p her make preparations for a sanitary place if there wasn't one for that baby to be bo'n. And we'd make pads to protect the bed and all like that. All a that come under visitin's I'm supposed to make befo the baby were born. Not all the time would it be sanitary. It just wasn't sanitary. Some a those houses were filthy. I told em it had to be sanitary befo I could deliver the baby in there. "Unh, unh, I cain't deliver a baby in here. You gonna have to clean this up. I'm not allowed to deliver in here." The Boa'd a Health nurses too, they came to visit just like we did. It's got to be clean. It's got to be real clean or that baby cain't be bo'n here. It's got to be sanitary. Some of em didn't listen and we just did the best we can. In fact I have went to a many, many places and carried my sheets and put on their bed. I ain't talkin bout all colored. I've carried em to white to put on their bed. The other chil'rens that was there, smaller chil'rens, they would urinate all in the bed and there was all a that. All a that smell and all a that. That had to be tended to. The Boa'd a Health went there too befo I delivered the baby. It was their job to tell em as well as it was my job to tell em that they had to clean up.

That is one reason they should've kep hangin on to the midwife cause we had a program that we have to visit our patients to see to them keepin things clean. To see to them havin things clean. That was our job to go and he'p make the proper pads that she supposed to get confined on and then change those out. You make one big one that they would get confined on and around three to fo to five lil ones that you change her every time you change her Kotex. She'd put a fresh pad on. That pad's supposed to have a sterile piece on it. That's for the po person mostly that's not able to pay these hospitals. All you got to be is taught how to keep that home clean. We was taught how to scrub our hands just like the nurses do, just like the doctors do. Indeed you've got to scrub. We had a program. It was a good program. Even at the last the Bo'd a Health they require the midwives to go out and he'p that mother that's expectin to get everything clean. Teach her how to do it if she don't know.

It was rough in those days. Much rougher than people have any idea and so many people then thought nothin about it. The fact was they had nothin. Fathers, the ones that did have jobs was small jobs makin such a small amount. When I first started fillin out my bedside books I put laborer down as the husband's occupation if he had a job. That's what I's told to do. Because they wasn't workin in no office and they didn't own nothin.

They wasn't workin in nothin like that. They wasn't no schoolteacher. They wasn't no prinicipal. They worked wherever they could make a dime. Hard labor, that's my point. There was plenty of parents where father wasn't workin at all. I delivered a lot a babies, that mother had three or fo and five babies or mo already and they would continue babies with no work and mothers didn't have a job. Even if a mother had a job it was makin around a dollar and a half, two or three dollars a week at most because I can remember when I came to Mobile myself.

It was just horrible for all these babies to be bo'n, some with fathers with no work and some with no fathers at all as well. A lot of em had babies and their husband lef after they were pregnant, and it was his pregnant a lot a times. They just let the devil get in there. That happens so many times. The mothers all had a hard time. A lot a times she didn't know where the father was. He was just out. He was not even workin, just wanderin around tryin to think where can I get a lil money to take home and then some of em wasn't carin whether they was home or not. Some of em were just playin around, that's true. When the father came home he found the baby and naturally they would put on a scene that they were so proud of their baby and glad to have their baby and all. At home they always act like they glad to have another baby but a baby at home wasn't the answer. He didn't have anything to give it.

When I walk into a house and find all a that where they have so many kids and cain't hardly support em, I'd wanna cry and plenty time I have cried. I did everything I could for em. I would clean up the house all the time. I would he'p em to wash. I would share my soap and all a that with em if they didn't have any. I would go in there and clean it up. I said I got to get this straight befo we can go ahead. I just clean up. Sometimes they didn't have nothin to put on the baby. Mother didn't have anything to put on the baby—had a receivin blanket. And that's all. Between contractions I would take an old skirt and make somethin for that baby to put on when it got here. I would sit there and sew it while waitin on the contractions to pick up. Cut it out and sew it and have it ready for something to put on em. In those days the girls didn't use Kotex. They used old shirts or old skirts to make their Kotex out of because they wasn't able to buy em. We was taught how to sterilize em and have em ready when that time come. We had a basin that was given us from the Boa'd a Health that we boiled our scissors and all in.

We was taught in class that they didn't want babies sleepin with mother and daddy. They wanted that baby separate when it was an infant. They wanted that baby in a bed to itself if we had to get a dresser drawer and put a pillow in it. A pastebo'd box if they didn't have a bed. We in our classes was taught how we could fix the lil box. And how we could do and line the dresser drawer. Mostly what I did was got a lil pillow for a lil mattress and put it in the box. Put a lil sheet over the box then put the pillow down. And when you put the pillow in the box then you get yo lil ruffle from the lil sheet all the way around. When parents they get sleepin there's been a lot a babies that got squashed to death. I've heard of it and know it happens a lot a times. Parents get sleepin and just forget about their lil bitty infant bein in the bed with em. That was the reason for that. There's been a lot a cases where parents had to use that infant-size bed. That pastebo'd box. Also in that time they had cane-bound chairs. Straight chairs as I would call em. You put two together like that and there's a cute way that you can put a sheet around it and put a pillow between there. Then you've got a lil bed. And I've done that so many times. Black and white.

When I went home after delivery I would carry whatever needed back. Food, soap, sheets, clothin that I could make. I would sit down a lot a days and just make not only the lil baby somethin to put on, the other babies too as well somethin to put on. A lot of em was hungry. A lot a times they didn't really have hardly bread for the lil ones in the family that was there in those times. I didn't have hardly anything myself. I was just beginnin to grow up on my feet myself but I shared whatever. I helped cook and he'p clean up. I would get breakfast and dinner. I did that all through the times with both my white and colored families. Whatever they needed and whatever had to be done I did it. I could just see Mother in me doin those kinda things. I could just see Mother all over and I still can see her. When I get to doin somethin that's constructive like that for somebody else that's what Mother would've done herself. That's what she wanted me to do. So I enjoy doin it. I'm workin for them and then end up havin to pay them. And I enjoyed doin it.

But anyhow, honey, you wouldn't want to believe what was happenin durin that time. Right here in Mobile. Downtown Mobile. I'd see some of everything. I know you don't understand two-thirds of it. I don't understand it but I always say God always made a way for the fool. He fed it. He put a lil piece a clothes on his back. He give it a lil spread. They survive one way or the other so it wasn't man makin em survive. They made their cover outa whatever they could get— old overalls and old this and old that and rip em up and patch em together and pad it with rags and tack em together. They did the best they could. God take care of em. It happens and they didn't know half the time how it happens that they would get a lil somethin to feed those chil'rens. It is just what happened. There is an old sayin which is true. You don't know where the next piece a bread comin from when you eat the last piece a bread. It happens.

I started repo'tin some a the families to Welfare durin my second ten years. Comin into my second ten years. Whenever I need to repo't somebody I didn't hesitate. I'd repo't. But if they needed somethin, food or somethin like that, I didn't wait to repo't that. I went and got that. I would get breakfast and dinner and then I know that no money comin in between breakfast and dinner. I had been in the kitchen and they didn't have anything and then the mother told me and I could see they didn't so I would carry the situation to the Boa'd a Health and the nurses would go out and see. I didn't start doin that right off because I didn't know to do that or how to go about that right off. But as soon as I learned and as soon as it was, I did it. You live and learn.

If I found an emergency—no food whatsoever—I'd repo't that to the Welfare myself. If it was not an emergency but they needed he'p I'd repo't it to the field nurse of the Boa'd a Health and she would see to it that the situation was helped. I've helped so many black ones like that. There was so many families I had to do this. When I went to deliver the baby they didn't have anything for breakfast that mornin. They wasn't any jobs and they just didn't have any money. I went to the sto. I went to the sto and bought em breakfast and brought it back. After I bought it I cooked it and fed the chil'rens cause he wasn't there. He was gone. He done got up and got gone tryin to make somethin. I cooked it and fed the smaller chil'rens. I went on to my home and took a bath and changed clothes and headed right on out the do' to the Welfare. My heart went out to em. They was so many lil bitty chil'rens. I said they need emergency he'p right now. There's several chil'rens in that house and those chil'rens are hungry. That ain't the first one, honey.

And then a lot a these mens, some of em be so sorry. If they made anything they did away with it befo they got home with it. I've known men as a whole, they would work and the wife would have the baby. Several of em had gotten paid off the very day that the baby come. There wasn't food in the house and he would stay out after his paycheck and get rid of all that. Here he'd come in with a brand-new baby and other small chil'rens with nothin to eat. I would repo't that. I repo't it to the Welfare and those nurses that work in the field. They would go from there. It wasn't so much that they would try to get some food for the family but they carried that man to co't and had him to carry his money down there too. He would have to repo't every payday down at the co't and then she could go get her money. That's how a lot of em got support for their chil'rens. And that happens now. They have to take that money down after they have a trial of it. The judge would tell em, "I want you to bring so much and so much every payday here. Bring it here and then she can go get it." They goes and gets it.

I saw plenty of broken homes, honey. Plenty of broken homes for thirty-eight years workin in the field every day. You might say plenty of broken homes. I have did a whole lot a ministerin to those broken homes.

But now let me say this about that Welfare. They way they distribute it, they didn't investigate enough. They hadn't did anything and they has ruint the ones that's on Welfare. They has ruint em completely. I've seen women sit around, young women sittin down waitin on the Welfare. Don't get up and try to get a job and do nothin. They waitin on they check to come and they spend two-thirds of it on their personal selves and the chil'rens be walkin around dirty, nasty, filthy and hungry. Right. Their chil'rens. And they're a lot a times they're unmarried. I know girls right today that got two and three chil'rens who get the money with the food stamps livin on the flower beds of Eve and won't hit a lick at a snake—they don't know how to sweep up their own house nice. They gettin the government money and usin it wherever and givin their own self shots, takin dope, and takin the other money and drinkin it up and still the lil chil'rens that supposed to be gettin it is naked as jaybirds and dirty and filthy and hadn't had a bath in two and three weeks at a time and they're starvin to death. I ain't talkin about what somebody told me. I'm talkin about what I've seen. They use the Welfare money on the wrong things. They're indulgin em is what they're doin.

The people that's workin don't investigate it enough. They got the wrong people out there. I had a privilege to tell one girl the other day. I said, "Let me tell you one thing. Y'all got the wrong job because you just indulge these people. You don't go back and repo't it like it is. You don't do nothin. They should get somebody that really knows how to handle Welfare. They should put somebody out there to teach the ignorant peoples what's gonna happen to em the next time you get a baby. Give her a job and let her go to work and take care of her own babies if it ain't nothing but gettin out there and cleanin her own outside toilet." I have went down to the Welfare myself and told em. I've talked to the field-workers. I told em just what I been tellin you. I certainly did. They say, "Well, do you have any proof? We have to have proof befo we can do this and befo we can do that." "All you got to do," I say, "all you got to do is get up outa that office chair and investigate and you'd have yo proof. Go by there on Friday evenin or Saturday evenin and see how much dope there's been and how much whiskey there's bein bought and you'd have yo proof." Back then, when I first started workin, the Welfare wasn't built up like it is now and you didn't see all a that like you do now.

It was several years that I was workin befo I started workin with the white. Mainly with the white it was out in the country. Way out in Mobile County where I have worked is just as much country as anything. Way out on the other side of Baker Field way out Old Shell Road near the state line of Mississippi—

nothin but country. Pure country. And way out to Wheeler right on the state line of Mississippi—that way I deliver. All over Wheeler and Semmes and Eight Mile. Durin those first ten years I did babies out in Wilmer. That's a rural area. They like me out in Wilmer. They sho did—both white and black. Usually it was a farm situation. The white families in the first ten years were all nice. It was nice and honest. I reckon it was the script from God and myself kep em like that, I don't know. But they were just nice and honest as they could be. We were just like friends. If it was different it was hidden inside and it didn't get out.

You would have to be a very very evil heart with no feelin toward a person—I'm not braggin on myself—to treat me any other way because I walks in just like I walk out. Feelin the same way. Glad to see you. Make you welcome to me and anything that I could do all the time. That's just me. I think if a person would do that that's all it takes. I think I have built up a lot a people that would have felt that or showed different towards me if I hadn't've had the personality that I have. I always have a smile and somethin good to say. I just have it in me to do those kinda doin's. I don't have to hunt for it. I don't have to search for it. It's there. So far as havin any trouble, I really haven't had any trouble. Major trouble, white nor black, durin my deliverin. There wasn't any prejudice just like I tell you. I have wisdom and knowledge enough I could've seen it and I would've known it cause I looked for it and I didn't get it.

I would say that with the white families durin the first ten years it was financial. That was the lower people that was stayin home to have their baby in those times. They couldn't do any better. But it was not all financial. In the country the doctor and the hospital was farther away. A lot a times it was the reason that the mother had two or three lil chil'rens that she didn't want to leave.

Yes, now there was a clinic when I started workin. They had a clinic then. They've always had that MIC [Maternal and Infant Care] clinic for these po peoples. Some of em just didn't take time to go to the clinic. But now I'll tell you the truth. The black people would always prefer a midwife. That's all they ever had and that's all they ever wanted. That's what they have always known. They didn't go to no clinic to have no baby. The general run of em was white that was runnin that clinic. The black have always avoided the white. Why? I can tell you why black people was afraid of white doctors. They was afraid for the way they know they was gonna be treated and talked to. They was afraid of — they knew how they was gonna be treated. Scornfully. They knew how they was gonna be talked to. Like they wasn't a human bein. They knew how they was gonna be treated and talked to. Cause there would be white in the hospitals and they were black. They knew how they was gonna be treated. So rather than to come down and be treated like that at the hospital, they'd rather stay home and do what God say do. When yo time come upon you, you out and get the midwife. That's in the Bible.

They was afraid, honey. Yes, they was really afraid. I know a long time ago black people were treated so dirty and so they was afraid of doctors givin em a dose of somethin just because they was black. They had that in their mind. And from the way they were treated, they had a right to think of such. They use the old sayin, use that word, they may give me the black bottle. That's the word they used I think. Means poison. Somethin like that just to get rid of em. They was afraid a that. That's right—they was afraid a that. Long years ago. They was. You know what? I didn't think nothin about all a this until—all a this really didn't dawn on me, plenty of it, until I just stopped and thinked. Then you realize it and you know it's true. They thought the doctors would do some kinda experiment on em. Removin this and removin that cause it wasn't nothin but a black body. Overall that's the way they felt. And I can see the point. But now it has been some time since they actually felt like that. It has been a change, you know.

Along about in that time I wasn't chargin much. Plenty didn't have any money to pay me. I said, "Well now don't worry. Where there's a will there's a way." I said, "We should have the will and God got the way." Over and over again. And plenty of ways it come up, sho did. When I was so nice about it, plenty have said, "I wouldn't miss it for anything. As soon as I get it." But it's got to be that person that God has had a lil dealin with their heart. They said, "I'm gonna give you two dollars now. Or come back week after next and I'll have it. Or come back next Saturday and I'll have this." When they got paid or what lil they were makin, plenty or most of em, the general run of em will share with you. They share a lil this week and next week they might not share none but they'll do it the week after next. They could tell me, "I'll bring you such and such" or "You can come by and pick up some two weeks later I'll give you a lil bit mo a this." I understood it like that. Both races would did me like that durin my first ten years. They would cut it two parts or three parts if they didn't have it.

I got about ten dollars for deliverin my first baby. In the beginnin when I was first startin to deliver I believe it was ten dollars. Thirty-eight years ago there just wasn't a lot a money. A lot a times we didn't get that. Plenty times I got nothin. They would dodge and wouldn't pay. I don't know whether they would have that lil that they could and just didn't. Sometime they tell me to come and I would go there and knock on the do'. They not home. They tell the chil'rens, "I'm not home." I always had to go back and try and collect. Go when they tell me to come back. "You come back next weekend my husband will get paid off." "I got to buy this and we've got to have a lil food to it." One thing or the other. "What I have I share with you." I had all those kinda words. They'd tell me, "I dudn't have any money but I'm lookin to do this and I'm lookin to do that and as soon as I start makin a lil money I'm gonna pay you." And I did with all these and thought nothin about it and it worked. That was not what was impo'tant to me.

When I first started I wasn't makin no money and I didn't grow up like the doctors. No money or money I did that baby. You might not be able to pay me a dime and I'll deliver yo baby if you're not able to pay me a dime. I was glad to do it. I was glad to be able to do it. Whether there be anything in it or not.

You know why? I love the work. I love to look at the work of God. I love to see the work of God. That is the work of God when you see a baby comin through the birth canal. You know man ain't doin that. It's got to be the work of God. It's a miracle. It's somethin to see. You will enjoy somethin that you won't never forget. It's really somethin to see. I've seen it so many many times. As I told you I'd rather see a baby born in the world, the different angles and the different things about it, than to eat when I'm hungry. So it's not a matter that I love to do it for the money. A few years ago it wasn't any money. It was just a lil change that you was gettin. Wasn't enough for to buy gas to drive over there. At the same time God made it possible for me as fur as makin a livin. I had other ways to make money for a livin.

All at the same time when I was deliverin babies at night I was workin full-time for the Mearses, livin on the place. Their maid full-time. I hadn't wasted a minute. I already had calls comin in as much as I could say grace on. Sometimes two a day. I've had one time three in one day. I've known one doctor to tell another doctor, "See that midwife over there? She's delivered mo babies in the run of a year than any doctor there is in Mobile." I hadn't wasted any time on my life.

Mrs. Mears loved to have big parties. She loved to have big plans. I was a good cook. I ain't talkin bout just fried chicken and easy. I'm talkin bout from the gourmet magazines. Because that's where my beginnin of really bein a good cook, makin all those different things, doin all that different kinda work, I was workin right in her house. She started me on all those major cookin's and things. She would give me recipes. "Onnie, I want you to make this. I want you to try to make this, see if you can make this now." She had all kinds of cookbooks and she'd fine one recipe what she'd want me to have. Especially doin parties and things like that. And I come out to be one a the top cooks.

I he'p her polish her silver, arrange her flowers, iron her linen, wash her crystal. She got so much a that you wouldn't want to believe—silver and china and whatnot. And the antique furniture. She got a huge flower garden. She loved her garden. So you see what I mean when I say I wasn't out there doin all that night work deliverin a baby just for a livin. For what was in it. I was doin a great ministry in the sight of God.

Dr. Mears thought my work as a midwife was wonderful. When I got my first permit I kep tellin him what I was doin and how it was comin out and he was so interested cause he loved doctorin. He loved to listen to my stories. He loved for me to sit down and talk to him about my work. Dr. Mears always thought I was very smart to take it up and very smart to do it— all the things that have happened to me durin my deliveries. He said, "Onnie, you would have made a good doctor."

It was understood by the Mearses when I got my permit if I walk in here to go to work and they call me in the middle for a delivery I'd sho turn around. If I walked in the do' and I got call I just turned short around and went back. It hasn't happened not a whole lot a times but it has happened several times right in the middle of great big dinner parties that I was supposed to serve. I had to walk off and leave the Mearses. Huge dinner party. It was buffet style and I had to walk out on that just as they was started servin. I was there servin and passin the plates at the tables. And I had to leave. Thank goodness the minute I walked in almost the baby was born. I was lucky enough to get there that when I walked in the do' the baby was born and I got back there in time enough to finish. I got through right quick and went on back up there because they wasn't but one back he'p. It was two or three times there was a dinner party at the Mearses that I had to leave for a baby. They didn't mind cause it was understood. I haven't had any trouble with Mrs. Mears. Not any trouble at all. I've never had—this is what I said befo—I never had as much trouble outa the Southerners. Mrs. Mears that I worked for fo'ty-odd years is the example. Hadn't never had Mrs. Mears to talk to me or treat me like I have been treated by somebody that's not a Southerner.

I do believe that it was meanted by God for me to deliver babies and to he'p the people that I have helped. There was this one night, cold and rainy, this boy had to walk about six miles or mo to get me in all that cold rain. This was after I had done moved off the place and had my own house then. So the police walks up to him and he's in all that rain and wanted to know— this is what the boy said he says, "Boy, what in the hell you doin out in weather like this?" Black boy. White policeman. Said, "I'm goin to get the midwife for my wife. She's fixin to have a baby. Would you all mind takin me up there?" And so they brought him over to my house and they were nice enough. They waited until he got knocked on the do'. Must've been about two or three o'clock in the mornin. He knocked on the do'. Then I answered it and he told me who he was.

They was gonna carry both of us back see, but I had my own car and I told him he could wait on me or he could let em take him on back and I'll be on. I said, "I'll tell you what do. You let em take you on back and I'll be right on so you can be there with yo wife." So he did that. They went and carried him on back. And when I got there—cold. The lil room that they was in to have the baby was in the back of somebody's else's house. They was livin in a lil room right next to the kitchen.

The only heat they had was a lil stove. I mean a cookin stove with the eyes burnin on top. Cold, cold. I delivered the baby and got her all wrapped up. The next mornin whoever they bought the stove from come to pull it while I was there. That's all the heat they had and it was still rainin and cold and sleetin. And I was there. And they was gonna take it. I said, "You move that stove outa here I'm gonna have you arrested." And "This new lil infant just been born here," because they was givin me the hard way to go. I tried to be nice you know and ask em not to get it. And they gonna take that stove outa there any ole how. And that's all the heat they had. They'd've froze. I said, "You go get that stove outa here I'm gonna go call the law on you right now and I'm gonna have you arrested for takin all the heat from these po people that they got." And when he saw that I actually meant that too. Was gonna take that stove outa there. I couldn't blame em cause I think they were doin what they were told to do. You see whoever sent em after it. So in the meantime they left it alone and said that we would give you another week—maybe the weather be better.

When I went back to see em about a month after, that stove was still there. I don't know whether or not he had caught up with it. I'm sho he had though. Found some money somewhere or another. It was tough then. It was rough to really pay for it so I don't know what was the consequences after that. That was about 'fifty-nine. They was just livin in the back of somebody else's house. They didn't hardly have their own nothin. She had three lil other chil'rens. Two lil rooms. One bedroom and the lil bitty kitchen. The chil'ren were asleep when the baby was born. Sound asleep. They was sound asleep durin the delivery of the baby but when those people come they was standin around the stove tryin to keep warm. Father didn't have a job. They had a lil food. Just barely any.

I delivered once for a girl that was about sixteen years old. I couldn't keep her father outa the house where I was deliverin the baby. I couldn't keep him out and I couldn't see the mother. Every once in a while I would see the mother. When it's cool she want the cover over her—all right. But when those contractions get close together they get hot. They don't want no cover at all. They want it off of em. Well this child had got to this stage and I couldn't get the daddy outa the room. He stood around in there and he talked. Finally I told him, "You're makin me nervous. I don't get nervous on my job. I don't like daddies standin around their lil girl. If this was yo wife it would be somethin different." So he went on out. There was a curtain hangin up at that do'. I was at the foot of the bed. When the baby got at the verge of fixin to come through the birth canal she got the urge to push. I said, "I'm go'n let you push just a lil bit. I don't want you to push much because I don't want you to clamp the baby down behind the pelvis." Finally when she got a good hard long contraction the baby was fixin to crown itself. I said, "You can give it a lit bit mo now if you want to. Not too hard. Just a lil bit mo." I looked around. That curtain was divided and he was standin there. You know two curtains come together. He was standin with his head stuck through the curtains like this. "Push, So-and-So, push," he says. I walked away from that girl. I said, "Let me tell you one thing. You may be the daddy but I want you outa here," because I was beginnin to put two and two together. So no mother. If she wanted a drink a water or somethin she would call Daddy.

So it rocked on and rocked on. I didn't have time to tell him no mo. When the baby started gotten through, the head like that, he was standin right at my back. After all a me insist that he got outa there he was standin right at my back. I delivered that baby and I told him this. I said, "I've never had a daddy that wanted to see a baby born so bad as much as you did in my life." He knowed then I was beginnin to put two and two together. Mother wasn't in there. Mother wasn't allowed to be in there. About that time when the baby were born I looked out the window. I saw him goin by the window. The baby done born now. He'd seen what he wanted and he gone.

I got through and cleaned up and everything. Myself and the mother went into the kitchen. I said, "Let me ask you somethin. What's goin on around here?" She said, "I know that you'd catch us. That's the daddy and the granddaddy. That's the daddy and the granddaddy." I said, "That's yo daughter?" "Yes, and it's his." "You birth her in the world?" She said,

"Yes." She said, "That's why I didn't come in. I had just been asked not to come in." I wanted to put him under the ground. Not in jail but under the ground. That's right. I couldn't keep him out and you know what? That's the onliest thing that I know of that really makes me furious every time I get to thinkin and talkin about that I get furious. Sixteen years old. That's the onliest case I ever run across of that kind but that goes on a lot. I've heard of it. The girl was happy as she could be cause she could call Daddy every time she wanted somethin. If I wasn't able to do it she would call Daddy. I said, "Let me ask you this. Why is it you're callin yo daddy so much? Isn't that yo mother? Why don't you call her? What's wrong around here?" That's exactly what I asked. Makes me so sick. She didn't tell me why. She didn't have an answer. Mother was indeed hurt. She was hurt. She told me. We went in the kitchen and had a cup a coffee.

The next day I went to see that baby—I go back the next day. By all means I go back the next day because after you tie that cord from birth, about the next twelve to twenty-fo hours it done shrinked and a lot a times it leaks from the stomach out. You need to retie it in the same place. So if it's gonna need it at all it would be durin the twelve or twenty-fo hours that it need to be tied tight. After delivery I stay two hours with the mother. Two hours after the mother had delivered to make sho mother and baby got settled and everything's all right. So anyway, they was livin in an apartment. The lady that lived next do' was on the po'ch just to tell me what had been goin on. The people that knows em well. They knew. She just asked me did I know it. I said I caught the hint. I did. I couldn't keep him outa that room to save my life. If I had known exactly I would have known what to tell that buddy and I've have told him. This was a black family. It's been a long time ago. Sixteen or seventeen years ago. Right down in the heart of Mobile. You just don't know what it did to me. I didn't tell the Boa'd a Health because nothin they could have done about it. It happens so much.

Now these young girls, fo'teen and fifteen year-old girls, can have a baby much better, as well or better than the ones in their early twenties, in their late twenties. I'm not kiddin you. I've delivered em. I'm gonna tell you exactly what I think. I think older men take advantage of these girls. I know that's what happened. It's not these boys in their age group and lil bit older. These are men which should be put in the penitentiary for life. I was thinkin a about her that she was young and she had that baby as beautiful as any patient that I ever waited on. She had a beautiful delivery and got along fine. No trouble. Just went through it. I wished I knew where she were. Fo'teen years old.

Most a the times when there wasn't a husband, they were so young that Mother just taken over. She did all the answerin of the questions because a lot a times the girls was so young. They had to have support from Mother. The whole situation was not left up to that child. She wasn't nothin but a child. The mother stood in front a that. The child she didn't hardly have anything to say. What was to be said and what was to be done Mother had to do it. So that's the way it was with that situation. She just never left home.

Naturally Mother wasn't pleased with it at all. None a the parents had joy of her situation but there was nothin they could do about it. They talked about it. They talked about how girls are these days. They get so you cain't do nothin with em and blah, blah, blah, you know. The fo'teen year-old was afraid. Her mother said, "Now listen." She wasn't married. "I couldn't tell you nothin. You went on and got pregnant. You did that and you're gonna have it. It's yo situation and you're gonna have it. I've got no money to send you to the hospital. You be quiet and do exactly what you're supposed to do." She did. She took it easy, cryin a lil. Her mother cooled down. She was not in labor a long time. She felt it just for a second there. Two years later she had another one. One or two years later. Fo'teen months later.

The girls resent it and some of em admit that they were sorry of what happened but then after the first baby they right back and do the same thing. A lot of em don't raise em afterwards. Their mother had to do it. Some a these girls didn't want to be married. They wasn't ready to be married. But they always stayed in a married person's shoes. When they get of age, you know, some of em would get out on their own. When they get so they kinda want a life. Nineteen, twenty, twenty-one, twenty-two years old. It's just six, one-half dozen or the other that lived by themselves or had men livin with em. So Mother would have to have another child to raise and feed.

Those black girls will keep their chil'ren. The black keep theirs with the mother or with the man or boyfriend or whatever. But the white they would either give em an abortion or they will adopt em out. That's why they don't have their chil'rens on hand. They just handle it different. That's why there's not as many white illegitimate chil'ren as there is black. That's the reason there's not as many. I know what I'm talkin about. I'm out there. Now and then you gets hold of some black that would take the time to get an abortion. They just don't take time to do it.

I would always lecture to those mothers that had illegitimate babies all the time. Not that I was makin fun cause that's not me. I always try to he'p. "I told you to be careful. I told you what would happen. I'm sorry but now you got you a fine lil baby. You just got to settle down and knuckle down to it and try to raise yo baby like a grown woman which you are not." I told em that. I don't think they were afraid of childbirth. They hardly didn't know what they was goin into. They just accepted it as it comes and went on through with it. I told em what to do, what they had to do and what to expect, and the mother did too. "It's yo baby. It's got to come here and you got to bring it here. It cain't stay there."

I love to talk to young girls even befo it happens because I am counselor over the young people of my church and has been for years and I always stayed on those girls about what would happen. I would tell em that they should try to stay natural girls. Take their time and keep their mind focused on somethin else besides boys all the time. I tell em that if they would take time with their life, nature wouldn't overpower em to let em want to have feelin's with boys or mens. If you would laugh and talk about the good things in life and leave that aside until you grow up to it or get married you wouldn't be so quick to jump to conclusion with a boy or with a man that's gonna get you pregnant. The first thing you know you'll be comin up with a child. I constantly tells em that. "Stay in your own category. Laugh about school, about books, about this, and about that and don't be so quick to get so close to a man or let him get so close to you because nature has no control over itself at times."

I'd say, "Take yo time. You've got all the time to do this." I'd show em where they was cutting their happy so short. "You don't know what life is all about. Befo you know it you'll have one draggin on yo dress." I would tell em that all the time. I'd tell em, "You're in too big a hurry with life. You're bypassin on yo happy life thinkin you're gettin to the happiness but you're not. You're gettin into worry. You're cuttin all yo pleasure out. You don't know what to do with this baby cause you're nothin but a baby yo'self." I told em that over and over and over again. "You don't know what to do with all these babies you're gettin around here. What's gonna happen to em?" That's the sad part about it. These girls that kep havin baby and baby and didn't want their baby. They didn't want em. Just what they done to get the baby. What I think about em I talked to em and not to their back either.

My husband had a daughter, Joanne, that got pregnant. This were my third husband. I had Watkins that walked off and left. Then I met this guy Homer George. He taken up so much time with my son. All that made me love him because I always felt that Johnny needed a daddy. He needed that manpower so he got it from him. Finally he died after a long time. He taken sick and died. I was married to him about eight or nine years. Then after so many years I met Logan and married him and that's where I am now. Hereafter a happy marriage. Don't want it to be any better. In fact, James Logan, I don't want nobody to be no nicer to me than he is. He is wonderful. I tells em that— the young girls at my church. My husband is not a good-lookin man. He's ugly. He's a big, wide-nosed, thick-lipped ugly nigger but you know what? He's the nicest human bein that I know. I just set em off with that but I think they see my point.

This Joanne was my husband's daughter by a first marriage. That child is around twenty-seven or -eight years old, the child that she had. She had him when she was sixteen. She was not married. I tried to talk to her just like I've been trying to talk to all the rest of em. That's all you can do. Cause you cain't keep em in yo lap or in yo pocket. She denied it to the last but I knew she was pregnant from about the second month and I told my husband several times about it and he didn't believe it so I just let it slip until push come to shove and I know she had to have some prenatal care. So then I got behind him and I carried her to the doctor and she still denied it when you could see it everywhere. So finally the doctor made a picture of her and told her. This is the thing that he told her, the same thing that I told her. "Two people that you don't make a habit a lying to. You can lie to parents. You can tell a lil fib to em and yo friends. But yo doctor and yo minister, those two people you always tell the truth."

How could I tell? I could tell by ways that show. She get sleepy. She get lazy. She would sit around. Once or twice I caught her with mornin sickness. She got cruel on her lil brother. She got cruel with him and he couldn't say nothin to her that wouldn't make her furious. There was the two chil'rens that we raised. Joanne and her lil brother. She was cross and she was cruel and she was hard to get along with. She wasn't hard to get along with me cause she knew to mind me. I didn't take no sass, nothin like no back talk. She did not give me that. If she wanted to do anything of that nature she took it out on her lil brother. She didn't want to marry the father. I couldn't get my husband to believe she were until I carried her and had the picture made. That was the first of September.

The doctor said, "Well, Joanne, now you said you're not pregnant. Look at this picture. See there's yo lil baby"—and he showed her. Then she looked at him and he said, "You should never lie to yo doctor. I think you might have yo lil baby sometime in December." I said, "No she won't, doctor." He said, "When do you think she'll have it, Onnie Lee?" That was one a my doctors that gave my patients prenatal care. I said, "Durin the first week in October." It was born on the fifth. I kep up with her period each month and I know when she missed it.

I delivered the baby. I attended her at my home. Fine delivery. Sixteen years old. She did all right. The next mornin friends come to see her and she talks a lot like her daddy anyhow. She said to her friends, "Oh, I thought havin a baby was somethin but it ain't nothin." I got so furious at her I wanted to pinch her nose. It was a boy. We raised it until she went to Ohio with some of her mother's relatives. That baby must've been about five years old when she left.

Never will fo'get this. This was a white mother come from Semmes out there. She came to me and she asked me to give her daughter a miscarriage. I have been asked did I do anything like that. I have been asked so many times. I had a lot a calls. They get ahold of my phone number that I was a midwife. Some be fo and five months pregnant. And some just when they think they just beginnin or somethin like that. "I just missed my period." "I missed two" or somethin of that nature. "Can you do somethin for me?" I say, "If you wait nine months I'll do somethin for you." They would tell me, "I think I'm pregnant, could you give me somethin? Are you able to take care of it?" I tell em in a minute, "I will deliver you baby, yo nine-months baby. You carry nine months and I'll be glad to deliver but to destroy, I don't know how. I don't want to know how and if I knew how, I wouldn't do it." I've heard a girl told that she has given herself an abortion several times. She started to tell me how she did it but I just waved her out.

"I'm gonna pay you this, I'll pay you this, I'll pay you that." I said, "You could pay me a thousand dollars and I wouldn't know one iota thing to do to destroy that baby and I wouldn't if I could." I never will fo'get—there's a midwife. And it was my husband's grandmother. My first husband's grandmother. She was a midwife. I nursed her until she died. I laid her out. I dressed her and laid her out. Combed her hair. That was in Magnolia right after I got married. She died and you know what she told me befo she died? "I could make it in if it weren't for all the lil babies. I cain't get by. I cain't get by for all the lil babies." You understand? She could have made it in if it weren't for all the babies that she miscarried, that she killed. I'm talkin bout me sittin right there hearin her say those words. "I could get by if it weren't for all these lil babies." I know one thing. You couldn't pay me to destroy a baby. They'll never get in my way from goin to heaven when I die.

I think the Boa'd a Health and the supervisors at the Boa'd a Health thought in terms of some midwives was doin somethin to bring on the miscarriages. I don't know whether the Boa'd a Health suspected all of us but there was quite a few miscarriages durin the first years of my gettin started doin home delivery. They said there was quite a few miscarriages looked like uncalled for. They've taken licenses from much older women durin that time. They taken licenses from a couple that they suspected. And I don't know whether any of em was doin it or not. I know one thing—I wasn't. I just didn't deal with that kinda stuff. I know my mother wouldn't have did that. You see me and you see my mother. I have always kep God in front.

I used to get a lot a calls for female trouble. You can get the female o'gans outa shape. Your ovaries can drop down. A whole lot a calls for that. A whole lot a calls for that. From black and white. Mainly black. You know a lot a doctors will say the midwife can do all a that. They have said that when people go to em. The midwives can do better than I can. The midwife, that was a real goal for the midwife. Cause that used to be quite a few womens that would suffer with that. It did happen to em a lot a times. A lot a times there is a certain way you can pull yo'self that cause this trouble without havin delivered. Get up and down too much. And then there it comes. It's painful too. It's painful. Sometime a lot of em have to crawl outa their bed and get on their knees and crawl to the bathroom. They be so sore. And if they didn't do that they'd walk like this holdin it cause it's so painful. As the old sayin said, those kinda pains, when you really got a case of that, it's just as bad or much worse than havin a baby. Happens to a lot of em. Then just new to deliver it's easy for that to happen to you. You start stirrin too soon.

Mrs. Patterson did that once. Like to died. They had them five boys. I said, "Mrs. Patterson, don't you be too fast." I said, "Honey, you get them female o'gans outa shape you be talkin bout crawlin. You gonna have to crawl outa the bed to the bathroom on yo knees. You ain't gonna be able to walk just cause it hurts you so bad down there." Sometimes they have to stay on the bed a couple a days so they can kinda gradually get back in shape. Her female o'gans got to get set back in place. The baby was born there at night and I went there the next mornin and Mrs. Patterson had done got outa bed with all her clothes. She messed around there. When I went back there the next mornin she couldn't get outa bed. I had to rub her up. I sho did. Put a tight band on her. Real tight band on her. They lay down flat and I rub em up and put a tight band around em. Make em take a deep breath while I put a tight band around em. My mother taught me how to do this. As I was growin my mother taught me.

When they call me and tell me they have female trouble I rub some of em like that. That's the old remedy that the midwives and the old mothers used to do years ago. It still works. I make a poultice outa maybe a lil turpentine and carbolated Vaseline or the plain Vaseline that mixed up kinda strong will draw when it hit the skin. That's what I rub em with. I rub em with that. Then there is Vaseline, a lil turpentine, and my mother used to use this plain pure lard. Put it in a lil rag that she had and I've used it too so many times. Clean rag that she had boiled and let it get cool. Then put this mixture in there and then you wrap it up. Make an oil out of it. You make a long string ball off a that and stuck that up and you can just feel it draw. You push it in the vagina and let em sleep with it at night and it's long hangin out like that, you know, so when you get ready to pull it out you just pull it out from the string. It works. I do that so many times to all of em. These kinda things in the old Indian remedies. We usually give em a douche. Vinegar, you usually give em a good douche first and then you rub em up and then you insert this ball and then just let em lay there overnight with it if they are so sore and so hurtin with it that they got to stay on the bed. Fact is they can walk around with it in the kitchen, you know what I mean. Whatever they got to do with that ball there. It's not gonna come out cause it's supposed to have a bigger head and you push it in. It works.

Then I showed em how to get outa bed. I said, "Don't just pull yo'self up. See you're putting a strain on yo body. A lot a times you don't be payin no attention that you are strainin to get up." I said, "Bring yo feets outa the bed and put em on the flo. You turn yo'self around and bring yo feets out and put em on the flo. You get all the weight off. Don't just pull befo you put yo feet on the flo. To roll on yo side and put yo feet on the flo and stand up and then walk off. Straight befo you walk off." I don't get as much calls for female trouble right through now as I used to. I haven't had very many calls for female pains for quite a few years. I've had some. Used to be all the time.

I had one call already at home for me, she thought she had female o'gans out and could I come and rub her up and fix that. I had been up all night. Just got home. I had been up all night with the baby I delivered. I said befo I start to undress—cause when I undress and get a bath now I'm goin to bed—I'm goin right over here and see what she want. So I got there and I went in there and I start lookin. I said, "You said you wasn't pregnant." "No, my other baby's just nine months and two weeks old." I said, "I don't care if he ain't nine months old. You fixin to have another baby." She said, "You don't mean." I said, "Just as sho as I'm sittin up here you fixin to have another one."

For emergencies I always carry with me some clean sterile old sheets. Always fresh newspapers and that's it for the bed cause I know how to fix it right quick. I keep pads already made that I can use with the old sheets that I done made the cover for. All I got to do is to get em outa that suitcase I got cause they're ready. They're the same as my bag. I always keep a supply of things in the car. I always keep a supply of pads. And that baby was so tiny when it came, that lil baby come so quick and so fast in the placenta it come out. The placenta didn't bust. I had to stick my hand and get it out befo it strangle him. See he was still in the water bag in the placenta. I've heard that a lot a small babies will come out in the water bag because they're not big enough and strong enough to press and he'p mother to bust that water or bust that placenta. I went on and I did it. I got the lil baby right off. Right immediately. I said, "Honey, this baby's so little." I said, "How old is the other baby?" I knew it was just about nine months. Nine months and two weeks. It was so lil I just sit there and looked at it to die.

I got up and called the husband. I said, "This child done had a baby." He come on in there and he looked and the lil thing was gettin stronger and stronger and just wigglin. I sit there and wait till it died. It was so lil and the lil baby was so young, I thought for sho it was gonna die. I sit there. I said, "This lil thing ain't gonna die. This lil thing is gettin stronger and stronger." So I said, "Mister, you're gonna have to take this baby on in to the hospital." I said, "But I ain't goin with you." I wasn't supposed to deliver a baby like that. I could've had a good excuse cause I thought the child had just did too much heavy work and had the female o'gans. So I got the baby wrapped and it was too lil to put on anything. I bet you it didn't weigh two pounds. I wrapped it up good and put it in a lil box. Put me some hot water bottles around it.

So I drove him down there with the baby but I didn't go in. I said, "Now you tell em how old that other baby is. You tell em exactly that other baby is not quite nine months and two weeks old." I said, "Y'all ought to be ashamed a yo'selves." I said, "You should be ashamed a yo'self." I said, "This is awful." So I carried him on in there and he told em that he did it but he said it just come itself because we didn't know she was pregnant. They said, "Well who wrapped it up and who tied the cord?" He said, "I did it." They said, "Who taught you how?" He said, "Well I remember a long time ago a midwife showed me how." They said, "Well you sho done a good job." Couldn't be beat.

They kep that lil thing, honey, in the hospital, must've been almost six months befo it was big enough and weighed enough to come out. I wish you could've seen it. Cutest lil thing you ever seen and it smile. She said that she just hadn't started menstruatin. You know a lot a times it takes em sometime a good many months befo they start back menstruatin after they deliver a baby. She didn't think anything of it. She didn't think anything of it. That happens. It was just a lil bitty baby. I mean a lil bitty one. She couldn't get very big the whole time cause the baby was so lil.

Usually when they get pregnant one right behind the other, they didn't feel as well. Cause they hadn't built back up. My mother had em like that. She had some eleven months apart, twelve months apart, ten months apart. That's the way she had all of em. She did have a hard time. Ten months apart. That's hard on a woman's body. It is. Could've been why she had that stroke. And especially she didn't go to the doctor and get any treatments or any nothin. Wasn't built up for nothin. Other than those old home remedies. Those teas and things that they would make.

Mens are ready for their wives as soon as the baby come out. And I can see the point. They're ready for em. And to my idea, I declare, they ought to give themselves a week. I tell em further than that cause I know they ain't gonna go as fur as I say. I never will fo'get. I delivered a baby, I believe it was the third or fo'rth day after that baby was born, this girl called me and that's what she asked me. "How long do we have to wait?" I said, "Now I cain't tell you how long to wait. You just let yo conscience be yo guide." That's what I told her. I usually tell people I would at least give myself between three and fo weeks. It doesn't take that long. I just say that.

You can have interco'se when you're pregnant but not after a certain time. That's what the doctors say. Now I think, to my idea really, it could be done easily if you just, and most of em do, just control themselves. They just don't insert way up as far. That's what counts. Rough handlin. You've got to learn to take it easy. Think about the situation. And it's just as well, just as much good, just as much service.

This is another one. It was a full nine-month baby but it was such a lil bitty baby, it didn't weigh but three pounds. We're really supposed to carry em to the hospital but the lil thing was in good shape. It cried strong, ate real well, and it wasn't no lil fainty baby. If you got that kinda baby when they're lil you got to take em out. He was so strong, mother she cried and cried. Don't take him. I'm gonna see to him and then I'd stay all night and half the next day watchin that baby to see cause if any changes was made I was gonna take off with it. That lil baby came out to be a great big fine minister right today. It was a full nine-month baby but it was such a lil baby that I should have carried it to the hospital but it really was strong and fine and in good health and in good shape. So I just let it stay home and I watched it all night and all day cause if any change would have been made I would have had to take him in. But the mother wanted me to leave him there. I said, "I'll watch him but if any change be made don't say nothin cause I'm takin him in." That was the third baby I did for her. That was a black girl.

I only had one baby to die on me durin my whole time and that was a lil baby three or fo years ago. One to die in almost fo'ty years. The mother got so upset because a the contractions. When she started havin contractions she didn't want to hurt. The harder her contractions got for delivery the mo upset she got. She just didn't wanna hurt. She just did not want to hurt. All she really had to do was hush. This was at the last stage. All she had to do was hush. She was a hard pusher. She didn't want to hurt. She didn't want to give up to it. She wanted the baby to come on so those contractions would leave her. She says, "Get this goddamn baby outa me." And when she said that God give it to her all at once. It came right then. Almost two gallons of water and the lil bitty baby. Just so much water. And the lil bitty baby. It was a full-time nine-month baby, it just didn't make it big. I felt that lil heartbeat but I couldn't get it to cry. I worked on it and worked on it tryin to get it to cry.

The husband was standin right by me and see'd it all. He said, "Honey, this just didn't intend to be." Because he was lookin at this lil bitty baby. It couldn't weigh a pound and a quarter. He made me feel so good when he said that because I didn't want to have to say that by myself. He just opened the way for me then to give my expression about it. I said, "This lil baby didn't meant to be. It just didn't meant to be. Not this." I said, "You can look and see yo'self that this just isn't meant to be. There was somethin wrong from the beginnin."

So finally I called the paramedics for some oxygen. They came out and put that lil oxygen on the baby and kinda did as I did by the baby to try to get it to cry. So he says, "Mrs. Logan, we better take this on to the hospital." And they did. And he was so lil and tiny I knowed it wasn't gonna make it. It lived about three days and died. We got the heartbeat but we couldn't get a breath. That lil thing was so tiny, honey. I declare it could almost fit in the palm of my hand.

Durin my full-time work I believe I only had about three stillborn babies. That's all. One white and two black stillborn babies. I knew each time. It showed up each time befo the baby was born. When she called me and told me she was in labor, then she told me that she had a show. I said, "Put it on yo Kotex and save it for me when I get there and I'll see what it's like." She had told me it was dark then and I know what that stands. I was almost sure so she saved it for me when I got there. When I got there she was really in good full labor. Wasn't in no time befo the baby was down at the birth canal and ready to be born.

The husband, I taken him into the livin room. I said, "I got to tell you and I just didn't want to come out and tell you over yo wife. Yo baby is a stillborn baby." He said, "You sho, Mrs. Logan?" I said, "Yes." At that time the baby was ready to come through the birth canal. I said, "I got to get outa here. Get yo wife outa here because I'm not allowed to deliver a stillborn baby." He didn't know how to believe how did I know that that was a stillborn baby. I said, "I know this is a stillborn baby." He said, "Well I'm goin back in there and tell her." I said, "Well that's the reason I thought I would tell you so you might know how to break it down to her." So he told her. She taken it beautifully bein a Christian-hearted woman. She was able to take it beautiful although it hurt. The next hard contraction she had the baby to come through the birth canal. The flesh that was showin bust. So we called the ambulance and put the lady in the ambulance.

I have had one baby born deformed. It was a black baby. This lil girl was born in the simplest lil bag. Like plastic was over it and in there you could see this water inside there in the lil bag. So I carried it on to the hospital and the doctor there, I wished I knew who he was. I think it was one a the interns or a staff doctor. It was the General Hospital then. Now it's South Alabama. He said, "Onnie, you see that?" He took time to show me. "You see that water there?" I cain't remember, he either said that belongs around its brain or that's comin from its brain. It was in the bag. So they kep it in the hospital, evidently about three or fo months. It lived to be about seven or eight months old. Had it lived it would've been one a those kinda people that got the hump across the back. You see mo white people like that than do colored but this was a black baby. That's the only one that was deformed.

I had a lil black baby whose toes all were stacked on top of one another like this. This on top of that. Other than that, the baby was in good shape. I scraped that baby's toes and put a boa'd and a piece of paste over it and wrapped those lil toes flat and I let it stay like that for about a month without takin it off. Those lil toes were just like they were supposed to be. I'm tellin you, what God tells me to do, I do it. All of em were stacked on top of one another on one foot. From the big toe on then the next one and on. I spreaded em out and wrapped em and taped that down and let it go about a month and then all the lil toes was just perfect. Right straight like it's supposed to be.

You ain't never heard the biggest baby I had to deliver. Fo'teen pounds. Fo'teen-pound boy. Richard Eugene. That was a challenge. She was a big woman. Big mama. Not so big a daddy. Big white mama. Big fat white mama. She was big, honey, she was huge. She was up there in the hundreds. They do work slow. It was slow. A big baby works slow. Always do. The baby worked slow. I just kep workin on that baby. My heart pounds and everything and when that baby come out I tell you I want you to know I stood up and put my hands on my hips and I looked and I didn't want to believe and I looked. Fo'teen pounds. She already had fifteen chil'ren. That was her last baby. She was a nice person and he was just overaverage good. He drank a lot. He didn't stay drunk but he drank a lot. They was po but they wasn't trash.

Now she's the one told me that her sister-in-law had had a baby for a black man years ago. She said that the husband did not want that black baby cause he knew it wasn't his but he let her keep that lil baby until it was around two and a half years old. She said it was the cutest lil thing you ever saw. Much prettier than any of the other ones. So one mornin—he kep sayin it wasn't gonna eat none a his food and instead of the lady givin it up for adoption—she could've called many people to come pick it up—instead of her doin that she kep it around there. So one mornin he got the lil baby and told the child to come on and go with him and he carried her away and don't nobody know today what he did with that baby but he gave her a hint that he carried her down to the dark river and put a weight on it. I'm talkin bout what she told me outa the clear blue sky she told me that.

So finally, bout three years later after she told me that I had a chance to deliver for that sister-in-law down in Theodore. He was there and you know you could tell there wasn't happiness in the family. I stayed with her all night and delivered the baby and next mornin just out the light blue he said, "Let's go in the kitchen and have a cup of coffee," after I had cleaned up everything. He would hint all a this seemingly to see if I had heard it.

He went out and cranked up the car. "What did he talk about when y'all was in there drinkin coffee?" See they're both suspicious. I didn't tell her. I said, "We just talked about things in general—my work and how I been doin and this and that." I didn't let it touch her but she said that it was just in the family and nobody never did question or nobody never did say a thing but that liked to have killed me. He might have carried it and give it away and give it to who he supposed to but I just don't think he was built up outa that kinda material. He done what he came back and hinted he did. That just tore me all to pieces. She said it was the prettiest one in the bunch. I think mostly that was the jealousy part. It was so much prettier than the rest of em. They say she was the cutest lil girl you ever saw in yo life. Now I don't talk this to everybody. The only reason I'm tellin you is you need to know.

Now I've delivered some half black, half white. There wasn't a whole lot a that goin on. Every once in a while that was happenin. I delivered for a white man and a black woman back in 1963. You didn't see a whole lot of it back in those days. Lot a people did like I did. They ignored em and took em as human bein's. I didn't think nothin about whether they were white or black they were just two together. I ain't worried, I ain't got time to worry in my mind about such as. Usually those babies of that nationality are the prettiest babies there is.

For the last I'd say ten or twelve years there's been mo white than there was black. Now I deliver mo white babies than black babies. There is a MIC clinic and the black usually go there. It's run by the government and the Boa'd a Health for the po black and white. The white families who engage me nowadays, it's not financial. It's not financial at all, not now. But then there's quite a few that say, "Well, I'm just not able to pay no twenty-five hundred dollars." If he maked too much money to go through the MIC clinic they tell em they have to see their private doctor. But it's not money all the time. Money ain't everything all the time. Money's good to have. You cain't get along without it but I'll be Joe Brown if it doesn't cover everything. A lot a happiness it doesn't cover. You can have money on top a money and be so unhappy it's pitiful.

I delivered Cooper's baby and you know he's mayor. He was the mayor of Prichard. They just wanted to have a no'mal delivery. They wanted a natural home delivery and that's what they got. He could afford the hospital but that's what they wanted. Mayor Cooper is a fine man. They wanted to give me a recognition. Cooper wanted to do that befo he left here in the auditorium and have all my chil'rens white and black.

Wouldn't that be beautiful? All my grandchil'rens. They sent me my ticket, my plane fare to go to Washington to deliver their next baby. The Bo'd a Health didn't know that cause I wasn't allowed to do that. I didn't supposed to do that. I stayed with em about fo days. God fixed it so that was one a the prettiest births that I have ever delivered.

Most white families who engage me nowadays are religious and don't believe in goin to the hospital. They really goes by the Scripture of the Bible. They want natural childbirth. They said that's the way God intended for em to have it. That's the way He intend for it to be. The Bible says when they wanted somebody to deliver Moses, they said go get a midwife. They say that that was an intent from God for home delivery. They wanna feel the pain cause God say for em that's what they were gonna do in the Scripture. It's in the Book. It's in the Bible. You should go forth and have pains. When Adam and Eve was in their garden, He said that Adam should make a livin by the sweat of his eyebrow. And she will pay for her sins in pain. Ain't that what He meant? All right now, why would man come in here and try to change that? Why would he come in here and try to change that? They put their belief in the Bible that God told woman He wouldn't put no mo on em than she could bear.

The white girls they start readin mo about havin their babies and they learn mo about what they do in the hospital. Now this is what they say. "In the hospital they acts mo like it's their baby than it's my baby." I'm tellin you what they tells me. I ain't talkin bout what I said. This is what they say. "I want to hear my baby when he cry. I want to feel it. I want to know what's goin on. I want to know what it's takin to bring my baby here. I want to feel it cause I know that hurt ain't gonna hurt but just so long." They don't like all that anesthesia. It's work havin yo baby at home without any anesthesia, but it's worth it. It hurts but it ain't sufferin. It is not sufferin. It's pain but it ain't the sufferin kind. It's a good hurt.

Mother knows the good that's gonna come outa this pain. She knows when that baby is born that she can sit up and play. She can take her baby on her bosom in her arms and play with it. She gets wide awake after the push comes and she get her baby and when the baby's born she's wide awake ready to play with her baby without any trouble, any medicine or drugs or anything. She's not sleepy anymo. She's ready for laughter. She's ready to play with her baby. She's got nothin hangin over her. They all with a happy face. They're not drugged. They'll sit there and smile and laugh at you and even the parents that's there or the friends that's there, say it's remarkable that she don't look like she's done anything. And that's true. They got the same color. They look so good, so rosy. My white girls they are and they're just reachin for that baby. In the hospital they don't get to see that baby for so many hours. God knows that's right. They done swirled that baby off in another room. The white girls say, "I don't want that happenin. I want my baby from the beginnin." That's what they say. I wrap my baby and soon as that baby is born I lay it on mother's tummy so that they could feel the warmness of the mother and mother could pat her baby. So many have found it out and that's the reason right now there's so many home deliveries. Especially in the white families. They have discovered that.

Hospital deliveries is a good way but now there's so many of em that'd rather not have it that way. I think they should let a person have whatever he wants. I don't think nobody should be deprived from what they think they should do with their own self and their own baby. Honestly, I believe a woman if she's in good health, I think she should be able to do what she want to do for havin her baby. That's her baby. I think she should be able to do exactly what she want to do if her health allow her to do it. At least give it a chance. It means a lot for a person to be happy and pleased over that kinda doin's. There's so many wanna stay home and be comfortable so they can enjoy havin their baby that they carried nine long months. That means a lot to the ones that wanna do it. And I think they should have the privilege of doin it without any interference.

Childbirth is not a sickness—God gonna take care of that. That's an intent from God. Now you do what God say do and I'm gonna do what God say do and you're gonna be all right. All you got to do is believe. God will make it work. He'll show you. I declare a woman gonna have a baby if she out there in the middle of the street. She gonna have it. All she needs is somebody to wrap it up and take care and put some clothes on it. Fact a business, she can get up and do that herself. If she lay there and relax herself just a lil while till that placenta pass she can get up and do it herself. Mother has her baby. Don't nobody do it for her. She's supposed to have her baby. Nobody supposed to pull that baby unless there is an emergency that she cannot have her baby no'mal. The contractions and the pressure brings the baby. Her pressure and her own sense supposed to discard that baby from her body. The pressure from God. God give her that knowledge. God give her just that much knowledge and that much wisdom. She can get up and do it herself. Just lay there and relax a lil bit until she get that placenta out. She can get up and tend to her own self and her baby. After she get up and tend to it then she gonna lay down and relax herself again. That's the truth as I ever told it. What happened then when there wasn't any equipment to be seen? My mother, I bet you she didn't see a doctor two times for sixteen babies. I bet you she didn't see a doctor two times. And it's the same God now as it was then.

Motherwit

To engage me they usually call the Boa'd a Health and say, "This is Miss So-and-So and I'm gonna have a baby. I'm lookin for a midwife and I want you to give me the name and phone number of the best midwife you got." That's the way I usually get the message. You know yo work speaks for itself. My name just got known through.

If we had a patient that engaged us we're supposed to let em know at the Boa'd a Health immediately so they could send a nurse out to visit em too. It got up to the point where we were not supposed to deliver a baby that we hadn't repo'ted the mother bein in prenatal. We should repo't her as soon as she engaged us. So the Boa'd a Health nurses made visits too. They'd go by and investigate and ask questions. See that she had her prenatal care and if she didn't have her prenatal care we wasn't allowed to deliver her. We had to get that one through to a lot of em because there's so many of em say, "There ain't a thing wrong with me." They just don't go. Most of em is tryin to avoid the cost and a lot of em just don't like to make visits often to the doctor anyway. First you have the financial part you might say. Then there are certain ones who will say, "I'm healthy. I don't need to go to no doctor. Ain't nothin wrong with me." Certain religions, mostly white, would tell you that. "God tells me what to do and guides me."

I always tell em that early visits to their physician is better for a lot of em because there is probably a lot a work that need to be done befo it's time to have the baby. It may take havin to build up a lil blood. You need a lot a counselin befo with yo

139

vitamins and all a that. It's better off for you as soon as you're pregnant. Start makin visits to yo doctor. If they get their visits as needed, it will he'p em to have a nice no'mal delivery. It has a lot to do with it if you're in good shape for deliverin yo baby. Now I didn't want to scold em but I had to tell em a lot a this kinda rough about takin their prenatal care. There has been plenty of em that did not take their prenatal care like they should have and then bring me my slip written up from the doctor.

I have to get on em bout that. Not hard but let em know that it was necessary and it should've been. "The Boa'd a Health requires it and I require it from you because I cain't do it if you don't get yo prenatal care and yo permission from the doctor that you are eligible for home delivery." I have done that. These are white and black. When push come to shove and they find out that they really had to go cause they had to bring a slip from that doctor readin such as "To Whom It May Concern: I have had Mrs. Blank in my office for exam. She's in pretty good shape or this is all right. Her back is all right and she is good and eligible for home delivery." The doctor had to have on that slip that he sent that any complications call me and I'll meet you at the hospital. That had to be on there because you had to have a backup in case. And that was good. Very very good cause you may run to the hospital with a patient with some kinda complications and no doctor. There won't be nobody there. So that was good. Real good.

I meet all my patients from three to fo different times when they engage me befo I deliver that baby. Rules and regulations were that we were supposed to make those pads and have things ready for that mother befo the time of delivery. Myself and mother together make the pads at her house. Do not wait until the exact time or the week befo. Make preparations. Go and visit em. Talk with em. Look at the bed. See how the bed's set up cause I cain't work left-handed. You have all that in front so when you got there you didn't have to start makin preparations for that. Good rules and regulations. Those was good.

When I go to deliver a baby I wear white. All white. My white coat. All white. We wears a lil white cap. That's a lil white cap comes around her tied to my head. It's mo sanitary than havin yo hair loose. I carry in my bag my scrub brush, my orange stick, a separate brush in a separate bag with my scrub brush in that. I sterile it when I get home and hang it out on the line to dry and don't open it again until I get ready to use it next time, my scrub brush what I scrub up with. The orange stick and the scrub brush is in a lil separate bag inside of the big bag. I have my sterile cord and silver nitrate and whatever to go in there is all sterile and wrapped from the Boa'd a Health. It's been sterile there and not to be opened until I get ready to use it. My coat that I deliver in, my gown, which has been steriled and pressed and turned on the wrong side. One side of my bag is my equipment such as my gown, my scrub brush, my orange stick. On the other side of my bag is all the equipment and stuff that belongs to the baby. One side is for my personals and the other side is for the baby with silver nitrate, sterile gauze, Q-tips, and all things that goes along with my baby when I deliver it.

I never have done without or been without my orange stick, my scrub brush. Not a single time since I've been workin. Now if those old midwives in those rare days didn't have any of that to work with I feel like they was doin the best they could. Got a job well done such as what they knew how to do. We're not supposed to carry any kinda medicine in our bags. We wasn't to do that. And we are not allowed to give any medicine other than prescribed by a doctor.

Now this is the way I did it. There was a beautiful setup with mother and daddy when their baby was conceived. They enjoyed it. When she get in labor—another beautiful setup. I think the husband and wife should be by themselves durin the first stage of labor. That mother and daddy is together quietly by themselves at her beginnin of labor until labor get so severe. Now this just comes from me. Even though some of em get kinda skittish and want me to come right on. I tells em this. "It was you and yo husband in the beginnin and it was fine. It's you and yo husband should be in the beginnin a the birth a the baby, quiet and easy, talkin and lovin and happy with one another. You don't need nobody there. Me nor nobody else until a certain length a time." That's the reason I tell my patients, "When you get in labor, you call me when you think you in labor"—especially the ones right here in the city.

"Let's have telephone conversations befo I come cause that's beautiful for you and yo husband to be together. Then every so often befo I get there you call me and let me know how you're comin on." And she will call me. Call me back in thirty minutes. Time yo pains and see how many you've had within the thirty minutes and if it be a good ways apart I says, "Well don't call me no mo until they start pickin up." We stay in touch with each other through telephone conversations. And when their pains start getting severe I say, "Well I better come on out so I can start gettin things ready." Once labor gets so severe that's when the two both wanna call somebody in that's experienced that knows what to do. I be prepared myself sittin ready at home so when they call and say they're getting rapid now, I'll be ready to just shoot out.

I look for the first two contractions befo I move to do anything when I first get there. See how they're percolatin along and then I start to work. Most of em, the general run of em have the bed all fixed because we done already talked about how and discussed it. We done made our pads three and fo weeks befo. Sometime two and three months. Pads for the bed to take care of the linens. We make the pads we can just roll all the ways in their clean bed. We made pads that big you know to take care of things like that. We use a plastic cover on the mattress and then there is a sheet on that. Then on top of the sheet we use these pads that we make that has been covered with a sterile old sheet. When we get through with that we just roll it all up. Roll it out from under her. Roll another one under her. And then she's layin there in a nice clean bed. No spots. The ones that hasn't laid the baby's clothes out, I get all a that. A fresh basin for the baby and a fresh basin for the mother so I can bathe her. Not in the same one. One for the baby and one for the mother. I have that all sterile and I go in and I sterile my scissors which I have a lil sterilizer to put on the stove and boilin water. I get all a that lined up. I time the contractions and I see how she's dilated.

You got some time now befo and I just leave em alone. I get me a book and get in the livin room somewheres in a quiet co'ner and leave em by themselves. I wait awhile till that time comes a lil bit later when pains get so severe that I get up to scrub up my hands because I got to scrub em up two or three different times befo the baby is born. Because we don't wear gloves. Scrub em up real good with a brush halfway up our arms. I did that through the rules and regulations of the Boa'd a Health in my trainin. They said that we could scrub our arms much better than tryin to wear gloves that we can't sterile. Of co'se we could use those gloves now that you throw away but they didn't have em when I first started workin. We was not allowed to go inside the vagina with our hands like a doctor anyway.

I tell you one thing that's very impo'tant that I do that the doctors don't do and the nurses doesn't do because they doesn't take time to do it. And that is I'm with my patients at all times with a smile and keepin her feelin good with kind words. The very words that she need to hear it comes up and come out. And that means a lot. Most a the doctors when they do say something to em it's so harsh. They already had contractions, and then with a ugly word to come out not suitable to how they're feelin. Some of em say that if they wasn't strapped down there they would get down and come home. A lot a women are left totally alone. And plenty of em have had their babies right by themelves. Well see I don't leave ⸱⸱᛫nt like that. I'm there givin her all the love and all the ⸱᛫nin it and they know I mean it. It's from my ᛫ feel me. You see what I mean? There's a lot of a certain lil black gal—they can feel that black gal. They can feel the love from her—the care from her. What she's goin through with I'm goin through right along with her.

Now I know how to stay away. In another room. Right. While I'm sittin right in here now, if you need me befo I walk back here you call me. I be right here. That's what I tell em and that works. And they like it. I'm right here. The most impo'tant thing is that I'm with em givin em love and care the whole time. I'm there from beginnin to end with smile, good words, happy words. Keepin you happy. And that's a very happy experience for you.

That baby works slow as I said. They work slow. When the mother gets severe contractions I tells her how to breathe. A lot a womens knows how because they've had a class. Now that breathin is just like a dose of medicine to the mother these days. It takes care of em so good and so much. It's so helpful. You have to breathe what suits you. It's whatever suit yo contractions. I he'p em find the way that suit em in their labor. I tell em when to breathe and when not to breathe.

Durin labor I kep em on their feet where in the hospital they buckle em down. I'd let my mother stay up on her feet until she'd have to lay down. Kep em on their feet and when they got tired and still in labor I would let her sit down and rest. Relax themselves. Then I know exactly what time to get em up. I know when they get tired they need to rest. That is a whole lot better than her layin there just lyin there hurtin. If she's up on her feet and havin contractions she don't feel nearly as much pain. They don't likes it when they have the baby, they buckles em down and the nurse and the doctors leaves em. They get so uncomfortable bein there and nobody sayin nothin to em and I'm right there to give em a word of encouragement all the time and tell em the way of life and the way of God. "Now look, honey—this will be over with soon, honey." And this is what God intended to do. This pain is intended to be. I'm tellin you so many of my white girls they don't fear. They reads up on it. They want to do it. They know what they be goin through with. They want to do it. They just set themselves.

I do all my work keepin em from havin lacerations and havin to have stitches. The doctor would've took her in there and give her a long laceration to get the baby. I had my own method of workin on those ladies so they could dilate. I didn't get it in class at the Boa'd a Health neither. It was given to me by God. I put em in a tub of water. Hot water. Hot as they can stand. Then they get on the bed, I get my basin and hot water and a towel. Just boil it on the stove. Make a lil sterile. Grease the mother with a lil oil. A lil white Vaseline real good. Then I start these hot towels. Just as hot as they can stand. And they say, "Oh, that feels so good. Oh, that hot compact make me feel so good." Because it's beginnin to get that burnin sensation where the skin has got to stretch. And that hot wash do good on em. Make em feel good. It eases em and it just stretches the skin out. And so I just constantly keep that thing on em. When that done cool off, not cold but just not hot, I'd heat it up again and put it back there. And they dilate so good without me doin any lacerations at all. Beautiful. I do that for everybody. He'p em to really dilate without needin any lacerations.

A lot a people wonder, "How do you keep em from tearin?" So I'm lettin out one a my secrets. I don't want to bury em. There's so much that I don't want to die with. Not sharin it with somebody. That's what give me the idea to do a book because I have so much experience in here that I want to explode. I was not taught to do that. God give that to me.

It worked. It worked. Now the onliest one that I know of it didn't work—that baby was in such a big hurry and such a big baby she forced it. You know you get to the place that you cain't he'p but push. When we got to that place that she couldn't he'p but push—that was a big baby. It was her first baby. It just come on through there. If you get it warm, greased all up, it will stretch for that head. But then there are a lot a certain skins that won't stretch either. That's the only one that had that big a laceration. She was Seven Days Adventist and they didn't believe in medicine. They don't like all this drugs that they give em. They try to go right by the Bible. They didn't believe in anesthesia. Nothin in that blood.

This was a white girl. The baby was born a beautiful birth. The baby came and she didn't have any trouble deliverin and everything was just simply beautiful. But when the baby started comin I couldn't get her to breathe and hold up. You know sometimes those contractions get so severe when that baby's head comes through the birth canal. A lot of em just give it all they got and that's what she did and that baby come on through befo she dilated good and just tore her all open. I said, "You got a big laceration." I said, "I'm gonna have to send you to the hospital to get some stitches," and they didn't at the time tell me about their religion.

Nobody but myself, her husband and her was there. So I got her all fixed up. I put her on a cot and he carried her down there and I stayed with the baby. Cleaned the baby up, cleaned the bed up, cleaned up everything, went in the kitchen and washed up all the dishes, was sittin down readin and here he come back. I met him at the do', the baby was sleepin. They came in and I said, "Oh, you all back." He said, "Yes, ma'am, we back, Mrs. Logan." She didn't say anything but she was he'pin herself to get outa the car. When I walked down the steps to he'p her up so she could get up, she looks up at me just befo she stood up in tears. I said, "What's the matter, honey? What's the matter? Are you hurtin? Didn't they give you no stitches?" He took it up. He said, "No, Mrs. Logan, I brought her back to you just like I carried her." I said, "They didn't give her no stitches?" He said, "No. She wouldn't take the anesthesia so they didn't do anything to her, brought her back to me." She looks up at me in my eyes and says this. "Mrs. Logan, me, you, and God can heal this." I said, "Yes, ma'am, we can heal it. Come on in, children. If you got that much faith you ain't go no mo than I got"—and I meant that.

I said, "Look here." I went on in and got her comfortable. I said, "Now you just stay right there and get a good rest and I'm gonna tend to you." I went in the bathroom, closed the do' after I got her comfortable, and I talked to God. When I talked to Him, He talks back to me. He told me what to do. Nobody had told me what to do until I went in there. Got on my knees and consult God and I come outa there knowin what to do cause He just guided my hands. He guided those lil hands and this mind and I did it and it worked. That give to know there's a high power somewhere and all you got to do is believe.

I did mo for that patient on account of her faith in me and God than I've ever done for any patient. I would stay night and day with her and keep her like I wanted her, like I was told. To do what I was told to do for her. I went to the drugsto and I got what God deal to me to get and I made me a squirt bottle. I kep her flat on her back. I said, "Don't you turn." Lay there with her legs crossed until I turned her over. I said, "You might get uncomfortable but I want you to lay right there." I would run home and give my husband his dinner. I'd say, "You stay right there, honey. I'll be back and I'll turn you over." And I turned her not too regularly the first thirty-six hours. She did everything like a child that I told her to do for almost three days.

So three years and a half later I delivered another baby for her and you couldn't even see the scar where she was torn and she was torn almost back to her rectum. I mean open. No stitches whatsoever. Yes. *My* stitches. That is the truth as I ever told it. It healed right back just like it wasn't there. The next baby she didn't have a scar. It was an easy delivery. No trouble whatsoever, not either one of em. She did not split the second time. You know the doctors don't believe that. They don't believe in it. That what I did was nothin but faith healin. And it wasn't all my faith. She had faith and I had faith and our faith went together. And it worked. With God's faith and with what God tell you to do, the doctors ain't got a chance when He want to walk in and show you He's God.

I declare to my soul, if God hadn't't've told me and give me all a this, I wouldn't't've fooled with the mothers and their babies. But I did and I learned to love it because I love he'pin a person. I'm just usin God's hands He gave me. I believe that if the Lord wasn't guiding these hands and this mind of mine that He lent me for a short while, I wouldn't've had that much success. He lent me these hands to work for Him. That's true. He just lent these hands. In all a my midwifin and all a my work that I do, I give God credit for. He guided me and he directed me in that. He gave me knowledge and wisdom along with a whole lot a experience. My faith in God is what carries me. A lot a people don't believe that the Bible says what it says. I ain't got no better sense than to read what it says that it meant. When God put the Ten Commandments on the rock of Moses that was enough for me. So I just went on from there.

Back in the days when my mother was a midwife they didn't do anything about lacerations then. What could they do about it? But I'll tell you why and what the score was with em. They kep em clean and they stayed on the bed nine days anyhow. That would make em heal back together—the grooves right in there meet the same grooves it was torn from. If you're gettin up you're makin it up either one way or the other. It will heal like that whenever it stick itself and that's not makin the grains stick together. Even if it won't buckle up it will slide by the grains that it's supposed to make connection with. Sometimes when it heals it don't even go back together. That makes her mo larger than she was. Makes her mo bigger. A woman she got to stay closed so that man can get the feelin between that. He don't want it so big.

As far as havin a laceration, nature's supposed to take care of that and it does along with me knowin what to do so she have a laceration and that's to use my hot towels and my oil. Be sho to let her take her time with her contractions and breathe and not push too hard. That's where the laceration comes from. When it gets to the point where she start dilatin beautiful, then she get to the place that she don't wanna breathe or cain't breathe. She get that urge to push instead of breathin. I tell em to stop if they get the urge to push. You gotta make em hold up off a that because they won't get through then.

I don't let em do it in a hurry. Just enough to give em a lil relief. Because you do mo harm pushin right now than you do good. You prolong the labor. See that baby would come down and get hung behind this birth canal, the pelvis right there. When you get the head behind that it takes a lot a long pains to bring the head up so it can come out. That baby's head got to make its own way. Breathe and let it come on down itself. Contractions will pull it. When it gets there it get that balance. That's when they can push slowly. I know when that point comes. You can only see the head. You see the dilation, a lot a times it stretch like that with the head back inside and that's beautiful. When you can look inside and see the head. You know then that baby is not gonna get trapped behind. Because you done dilated her all you need then and a lit bit mo pressure so it can come out. I tell em how much to give and how much not to give.

When they get in that last stage of labor they sometime get to cryin and start to say what they cain't do. "I just cain't—I done tried. I done all I could. There ain't no mo I can do." That is the worst feelin for the mother at that stage of labor. Mostly those contractions is the worst. I just tell em to leave the rest to God. "All I want you to do is be calm and easy." Plenty times I say, "All you got to do is hush yo mouth and you'll see it ain't worth the vibration you're makin, you'll be through." Plenty times I say, "You done had yo baby. All you gotta do is hush yo mouth and let me reach in there." They done had all the contractions it takes to bring that baby down comin through the birth canal. All they have to do is be a lil patient. Just a lil patient. You see who gonna handle the rest of it. I say, "Now right here is where God comes in. You say you done all you could. You done beared as much as you could. Leave the rest to God. He'll do it."

In the last stages of labor when the baby is fixin to crown, that's when really, you really get irritable. They don't want to be bothered and they easily get furious. Just like I had one girl, I says, "Well, honey, you're doin fine." "Mrs. Logan, you don't know what you're talkin about. You ain't never had no babies." Well that wasn't her. That was the stage she was in at the time, see. When they get in that last stage of labor just most anything they say would come up. And all at the same time the baby was crownin, it was comin out. I stay cool and calm. Don't you get irritable like they are. You got to know better than that which I do know better than that. I know better and I just keep my calm. Smile and say somethin to em. Finally they get right along with you. But if you gonna start actin up along with em and gettin disgusted with em—now that's somethin I have never: really got disgusted with a patient.

I ask em not to push at this point. Cause at that time they're right at that stage if I would let em start pushin, that would give em relief. But see I didn't want em to push right there. It just do a lil bit mo harm than good. When they get to the stage that they really cain't he'p but push, well I knows when that stage come. And they know it. And I say, "Come on, dear, push just easy, not hard. Don't give it all you got. You understand? Just push easy." And it works simple. So simple. They do, it starts workin right there. And they get relief from the pressure when they can push. But they're not supposed to push at some of the last stages. Just breathe. When they get that baby's head crowned, then that's when they're supposed to push. If that shoulder is a lil wider than the head, they got another stage there that they got to put a lil pressure on. And when they get that shoulder through, then the body will just slide out.

If you push too soon, instead of that head comin like it's supposed to you pushin behind that pelvis right there. Instead of pushin it so it would come out, it's pushin against that. As long as you push against that it's not gonna come. It takes a lot a pushin to pull it up so it can come. But if you don't push too soon it'll bounce right up and start out. On its own. I know exactly when to keep em from pushin too hard. Slow em cause some of em will be in such a hurry and want to get through with it. Cause they don't want to hurt. They want to get it behind em.

The contractions can leave awhile completely. That's God's way. That's what I love about it. Give mother time to rest between contractions. This is a beautiful point about it. They gets so sleepy just befo that baby is really fixin to crown on us yet, mother gets so sleepy. That's the anesthesia God give em. I know that's true. They can rest. I don't care what no doctor say or nobody else say. That is the anesthesia that God give mother. He said He wouldn't put no mo on em than they could bear.

And befo you think you're gonna give or it's gonna kill you, He take it completely away and make you sleepy. You cain't stay awake to save yo life. That's anesthesia from God. Man had nothing to do with that. It's true. These thirty-eight years that I've been workin it's true. God have deal it with me. I have experienced it. I have looked it over and over and over and God give it to me. That is true.

Some of em say this. "Onnie, if these pains would just hold up so I could sleep one minute I would feel better." God take it away. I don't care if they don't hold up for that lil length of time—they sleep just that quick. Just befo it crowns they get those hard severe contractions that they're not gonna be able to do nothin but push. Befo they get the urge to push that's when they get sleepy for a rest. That's true. Honey, when it get right to the last minute they think, "Well, I done gone as far as I can go. But God give me new strength." He will take the contractions away from em and they get so sleepy. He gives em some anesthesia between time. I've told so many people that. They looks at me and say, "Where is it you get that from?" I said, "God gives that to me and tells me to tell you that and it's true."

I had a hernia for years befo the doctors knew what it was. He'pin that mother with those last contractions. Makin her strain through here with these arms. A hernia come mostly from strain. Strainin in the chest from here usin these arms. They would be pullin on me or a lot a times I would be pushin em. The mo pressure they could put on me the better they would get relief. Not only relief but the work that they was doin would act. It would come better. It would dilate better if they had somethin to go against. I was just as tired as they were until I learned better not to bear along with em. Not to let the contractions strike me as it was strikin them. So I found other ways.

I have mothers that enjoyed the last pains so much so in the bathroom sittin on the toilet stool. When the baby could crown at any minute. It he'ps em. They get relief from their contractions to sit up on that toilet stool. That's a good place if you know that water gonna break in there without that baby comin with the water. A lot a times they come together. I said, "Why don't you go on back in there? Get back on the bed. You done dilated too much like that. Now go on back in there." "I just cain't. I got to urinate and I just cain't do it." You know the baby do press against yo bladder and make you want to urinate. I said, "Yes, you can." "Won't you please just come on and go with me back there just one mo time?" "I'm not gonna let you have it in the bathroom...Okay, sugar, come on. Let's go."

I always stay with em when they go to the bathroom especially when the pains get pretty close together. The water might break and the baby may come right there. I coach em if the baby is crownin while they're on the toilet. It was understood to em now if you get a contraction that won't turn loose while you're on there, I want you to drop to yo knees. Couldn't get em back to bed on account of that contraction. And I couldn't tow em back to bed.

I say, "All right. I'm gonna take you to the bathroom and if that baby start comin through the birth canal, you cannot walk back to bed. That's breakin the baby's neck. You got to do what

I say. Do you understand?" "All right, I'll do it, Onnie." She's sittin on the toilet like this. When I see that baby comin I say, "Breathe, honey, breathe. Breathe fast. I want you to drop to yo knees. I want you to come right on down and lean on the tub." I run over to the bed and pull all my paddin I had on the bed. Throw the pads on the flo. Nice comfortable bed for the baby to come. And I get behind em. Get down right behind her in the bathroom on the flo. I get the baby's head and get it on down and she is up on her knees like this. I say, "When I tell you to start sittin back you sit back." That's in order not to pull that cord from the placenta and the baby be too tight, you understand. So when she leans back, she go down fur enough that the baby is on the flo on the pad and the cord had a lot a slack in it. I say, "Now relax yo'self, relax." And she relax herself down. Then I run get the scissors and the sterile gauze and I tie the knot and I get the baby leavin her still hangin over the bathtub. Leavin her hangin over the bathtub. I went get the baby from the placenta and I leave the placenta with her. I run in the bedroom with the baby and wrap it good and warm and lay it there and let it stay there. Then I go back and get her. I get the placenta. Get her all washed up still on her knees over the bathtub. I get it down all on the paper. Pull all my paddin. No spots on the flo, no nothin. All right on that paddin I have all ready on the bed for her. And then I get her up and go and pad the bed right quick again cause I have another pad to put on her after the baby anyway. Put that on there and get her back on there, and she is just as happy. See how God works? I wished I had a flower for every time I did that.

There are so many women that want to have babies in that sittin position. It's not unusual. It feels good. Mother gets mo relief. Now it might not be mo relief for you but it will be for her. There may be another position that would suit you better. I have delivered babies on purpose on their knees like that with a chair like this here. Because that makes her comfortable. I had mine on my knees. It's whatever makes you comfortable. I will do that for a home delivery cause that's the purpose of a home delivery. That's the privilege of stayin at home. You let em do what they wanna do. You name it and I've done it. The doctors just don't do that. In a hospital you cain't move. You're so tired of layin that way and you get cramps in yo legs and then yo knees. That's how come women holler so when they're in the hospital. Their whole body hurts. That's miserable, honey. You think it's not but that's miserable to lay up there with both of yo legs up like this and you're layin down and you cain't move nothin but yo head.

I let em walk until their baby get ready to come through the birth canal. You walk and sit down and you walk. Try to make mother comfortable from these contractions. Let her do mostly what she want to do. That's the good purpose of stayin at home havin a baby. If you got a good midwife or somebody that knows what she's doin and knows how to watch mother and knows how mother's comin on, she'll let mother do just exactly what she want to do. And say, "Now I'm gonna let you do yo thing but now when it get to this point, I want you to do what I tell you to do." You tell her that between contractions. You don't tell her that when she's havin a contraction. And she'll pay strict attention. And it'll work out.

As I say, I let em do first one thing and then another. Sometimes they want to be first in the bed, first out the bed, in bed, out bed. Well I know the baby is not fixin to crown and that's good for mother and I just let her do it. Now don't get me wrong. I'm right there with her, watchin her, holdin her. Right at her fingertips for her. When I get em up to walk, contractions slow down, and see usually when the contractions start they want to hurry back to bed. I say, "Don't do that. Right where yo contractions start, a table or anything, just lean awhile until that contraction leaves. It's no use tryin to hurry back tryin to lay down cause yo baby ain't comin yet."

I have had some of my white girls want me to let em have their baby lyin on their side and I don't like that. That wouldn't work and I just told em in a nice way that wouldn't work. That's not too safe for the baby. I cain't protect the baby's neck on the side as well as I can on yo back or on yo knees. If she's on her knees I say, "Now as I talk to you, you do exactly what I say. As that baby's comin through the birth canal like that, squat back until I get the baby just gradually start comin out and then yo buttocks is close to the flo." The birth canal is close to the flo and then when the baby come I lay it down and get the cord out far enough and then she can pull back on her knees. Kinda come back up. It's easy and the baby's perfectly safe layin on the flo on the pad.

I do whatever is suitable for that minute or that hour or that situation. I do it. I do it. Whether I've seen it in a book or read it or not, I do it. And it works. A lot a mothers says, "I didn't do that with my other baby." I say, "That was that baby, honey. This is this one. They are all different. What I did for you then I might not be able to do for you next time. Honey, everything it changes. And you got to have knowledge and wisdom which comes from God on high enough to change with it. When it says do this you do that and don't think about what you done last time. I gave you that hand to do that then. Now I'm givin you another had to do this. This baby is different."

I've seen so many and there are so many different ways a baby can come into the world until I'll be lookin for a different every time. This is the beautiful part about it. When the baby comes, its face is down when its head get through the birth canal. A no'mal birth. The face is down like that on the mattress—down that way. But befo that whole body get out— you would think that neck is breakin but it be done turned and his face is up. It's beautiful. Some babies they don't get to turn all the way over. They turn from down on the side. Their face is on the side when they come. Then you may get a case every so often that the face sometime come all the way out and the baby too befo it turns over. You don't pull the baby. You just guide the baby's head. It a lot a times when the water and baby comes together right under the mother is maybe a puddle of water. I puts my hand under its lil face and head to keep its lil nose outa that water cause the head's gonna turn anyway. But you got to guide it. It's just a matter of guidin that body. All you got to know is how to handle it. Sometimes I see my baby with a cord around its neck. As long as I could get this hand between that neck and that cord, it's not gonna choke that baby. I've had it wrapped around his neck three times. If it's not too tight as soon as the baby is all the way birthin, I can get it out right over its head.

I had a black girl one Sunday morning, the baby's face was comin first. That's dangerous—breakin the baby's neck. I worked with that. It had to work itself out. What is this I see comin first? It was comin through the birth canal. It took me about three contractions befo I could recognize what it was. Her lil lips when she had the contractions and that's all I could see. Then it come to me about face first. That's what it was. When she had the next contraction it was hard and the lil face come first and then the lil chin was fixin to come and I know that was dangerous. I crossed her legs. I put her in my car and I hauled off to the hospital with her. The doctor told me, "You know what this is, Onnie?" I said, "What is that, doctor?" He said, "This is what you call face first." If that lil face would've come out first it would have just snapped the neck. He knew what to do. He said, "The next time when you discover, take yo fingers"—he told me this—"and run up there and feel for the cheekbone. The next time a contraction come you pull that lil head down and this will come first just like it's supposed to." I've had to do it just once.

I had one the lil hand fell completely out when she had a contraction, and this particular girl I had delivered five chil'ren for her and that was her last one. They had to give her a caesarian when they got to the hospital. The lil arm fell out after the contractions. Between contractions I put that lil arm back. I put that lil arm back and took her to the hospital. She said, "Let me try it again." The mother was just that strong she didn't want to go to the hospital. She said, "Let me have one mo contraction befo you take me to the hospital. Maybe the baby done turned itself." When she had the next contraction that same lil arm tried to come back and I told her, "I'm not tryin anymo. I'm not gonna let you have any mo contractions." It was one Sunday night. I never will fo'get that. They give her a caesarian and got it from the side cause the baby was crossways. That baby was lyin crossways. No way it could come out.

When the baby's delivered you wait so many minutes until the baby is getting whatcha call a blood transfusion from the placenta to the body. The heart is beatin through that cord that's attached to the baby's navel to the placenta. I usually wait calmly until you cannot feel that heart beatin through that cord. You catch it like this and when you stop feelin it through there you tie it and cut it loose and I usually tell my babies, "Now darlin, you're on yo own." You ain't on yo mother no mo from that minute on. That's what my sterile scissors are for. That's all I have. That's it. You tie two knots befo you get the placenta from the mother. You tie one bout an inch from the baby's stomach and then about two inches from that tie up the cord. Then you cut between there to get the baby from the placenta. I don't have to clean the baby up first. I get mother comfortable first because to get the baby comfortable is to get it out loose from the afterbirth and wrap it up so it could get warm cause he'll go back to sleep if he done gotten warm.

Then I get the placenta from the mother. Mother usually give slight contractions, especially the second baby. You want her to have a certain po'tion of afterpains because that he'ps clean the uterus out. Usually mothers don't have afterpains with their first babies. Now and then. And if they do, it's just minor enough to clean the uterus out. The afterpains usually start after the second baby. And then after the third baby, they're a lil bit harder than after the second baby. And the fo'th baby it's a lil bit mo. I don't know what that is. God aimed for us to know just so much and that's it. Because He's gonna take care of that part anyhow. Now it could be that it takes mo pains to clean the uterus each time or to make their uterus get back in its place. You see what I mean? Ain't God beautiful? Make me wanna scream on how it all works. There's a purpose for it. There's a call. There's a reason for all that. It's amazin.

Mother get a slight contraction and she kinda press it out slightly and the placenta come on. A lot a times it's not turnin loose from the uterus as yet so we just wait a lil while. I wrap mother up and go back and tend my baby then go back to mother and the placenta's ready to discard itself. That's the afterbirth. Take it out and open it wide and look to see if any pieces are left. Most of mine I examine real good to see if there are any lost pieces cause it's like poison, you know. If there are any left, you don't have to get em out, you watch for em to pass through the flow. If it doesn't pass then they'd have to go to the doctor or the hospital to get what you call a curettage. I had only one patient to have that to happen. If no pieces are left you roll it back up just like it was, then wrap it in paper.

They required me to get rid of the placenta, to burn it. Fact is, we was taught in our class to burn it. But then through wisdom and knowledge I learned better cause it takes you a long time to burn those things. It all depends on how much wood you have. It takes a long time befo it gets hot enough to start burnin it. It draws up in a knot and get just as tight. Draw up in a knot and get just as tight and it takes a lot a fire coal wood. Done burnt down to hard coal to start that placenta to burnin. It makes a big hard ball when it gets hot and it stays in that big hard ball a long time if you don't have wood. You keep it on a good base fire to get it to started to burn.

I never will fo'get, years ago when I delivered out on the south part a town one night, myself and another lady that was workin with me. That was when I first started workin. They wasn't as particular about fire durin that times. So right off the street kinda in the back, we had this big fire out there in the backyard. Must've been about two or three o'clock in the mornin. We were burnin all the trash. We use paper now with a cloth on it and we burn all that. So we were burnin all a that and had a big fire out there and the police stopped by. They come and say, "What's happenin? What's the big idea for such a big fire this time a the mornin?" "Just cleanin up after from deliverin a baby. You like to give me a hand?" And they walked on back. "No thank you. You're doin a good job at it." Sho did.

I was so glad when they got to the stage that I didn't have to burn it. If they have a shovel and a backyard, the husband dig a long deep hole and put it in and bury it. Then right in the city where they didn't have no place to even bury it, when they was livin in the projects, they didn't even have places that they could bury it. I wrapped em up in plastic and carried em home. You want to see me count the many that are buried in my backyard? There's a million of em buried in my backyard. A million, million placenta. A million placentas is buried in my backyard. I have peach trees and whatnot trees back there. I buried a lot a placentas around that peach tree. I had the biggest peaches you ever did see. Mo than I could sto off that one lil tree but Hurricane Frederick messed it up. After that, if I delivers like the mornin about daylight or befo, if the garbage man in comin on we put it in the garbage can if he's comin that same time. Or if it was like late in the evenin and the garbage men was comin on tomorrow mornin, we put it in the garbage. But you couldn't keep it there for a couple of days especially in the summertime.

When I first started to work as a midwife, a lot of em, especially white patients, didn't want you to do the silver nitrate. We put drops in the baby's eyes, the silver nitrate. The babies would look like somebody give em a black eye the next mornin after putting the silver nitrate in. Cause wherever the silver nitrate gets on that white skin it's just as black around his lil eye. My supervisor said, "Well if they don't want you to put it in don't put it in." Then the law took a hold to it. It's a law now that we have to do it. So one mornin befo day I woke up, somethin told me in my sleep. Next time you have yo white babies, get the blue-sealed Vaseline and rub around their lil eyes real good befo you put the silver nitrate in. When it hit it doesn't hit the skin. It hit that Vaseline. No mo black eyes. That's been years ago. I carried that back to the Boa'd a Health and they all did it from there.

* * *

Now they all liked me down at the Boa'd a Health except one. When I go to get trays and umbilical cord dressin's and all that I get from the Boa'd a Health, everybody just be so glad to see one another. But not Mrs. Camp. She's the one that's sit over there in that co'ner and look at me like I was somethin that stunk. She didn't ever say anything to me—just looked. That's the way Mrs. Camp treated me. She always give me those lil cuts. When I come in to have a meetin with Mrs. Pete or Mrs. Davidson or go in to get me some supplies, Mrs. Camp just looked at me like I was somethin. I know where it was comin from. I knew the whole time I'm sittin there waitin there was prejudice. And when they made her my supervisor I didn't let nobody know but I was disappointed within my heart. I never said anything to anybody about it. Because I could see it and feel it and I knew that she didn't care for me. And she has not spoke a good word to me since and that's been goin on three years. And you wanna know the truth? She knowed as much about supervisin there as you do. You know you don't know nothin about supervisin there. And she knew I knew everything and I knew five times mo than she knew about it. You know—let me tell you this. If a Negro shows common sense and a lil knowledge that God has sent down to her or him from on high and they use it a lil bit, then that's where the white get prejudice. And they say, "You're tryin to be smart." You understand me? And that makes em just stare and try to wave the bad thing out. Instead of lookin that we are people, we are human, let's join our life together and live.

Let me tell you somethin and this is the way of truth. If every white person under God's sun just was to believe it—if you cain't live with me down here we both cain't live together in heaven. Cause God ain't got no co'ner for you up there and another co'ner for me so we got to try to get together and live it right here. When the time come for it to be boilin down, you are my sister and I'm yo sister. We're supposed not ᵗᵒ ᵇᵉ ˢᵃⁱᵈ you're my black sister and I'm yo white sister. We ɑ

\

'ther you're black or white. The mo we live together
_ _iate together and communicate together, the closer
. ε will get as a human person and that's what God aim for us
to do. That's what He wants for us to do. You got to stop lookin
at my black skin and I got to stop lookin at yo black heart. I
want to clear up yo black heart and I want you to clear up in yo
mind about my black skin and we'll get together as a human
race. Instead of that you can just stand there and count
prejudice. Up to thousands. You can just look at it.

The police stopped me once when I was on a delivery.
There was a time I had been to an usher boa'd meetin. Church
usher boa'd meetin. They called me at the church that I was
needed in Mobile Terrace for a delivery. I was on my way goin
up Springhill Avenue in a thirty-mile zone makin about thirty-
one and a half miles an hour. My husband was with me. We
had been to usher boa'd and they called us at the church and
let me know that I was needed. So when I was goin on home
my husband said, "Honey, I think that's the police behind you."
I said, "Well, honey, I'm not speedin. I just got to get home, get
changed so I can get on out there. They called me. I got a call."

So he blow me down. And when he blew me down I
stopped and he says—he didn't say nothin. It was one a those
white that had a great stubborn attitude. Wouldn't say nothin
to you. If he did say anything, he almost cut yo throat. So I said,
"Well, officer, if you don't mind I'm in a hurry. I'm's a
midwife." I said, "I'm on a delivery right now and I still got to
go out to Mobile Terrace." He still wrote that lil ticket up.
Didn't say a word and he didn't say a one word to me. I said,
"My time is up. If anything happen to that baby and mother I

will be held responsible for it befo I could get there." He didn't open his mouth. He go on and took his own time and written that lil ticket and gave it to me. I went on out there and when I got there the baby was born and the baby was dead. Yes it was.

I taken that ticket the next morning and I went down befo the judge and I showed it to him when I went to co't. I showed it to him and I explained everything to him. How long I was held up to get a ticket written. You know sometimes it takes em thirty or fo'ty minutes to write one lil ticket. It look like they been writin em so much they oughta say chit chat chit and it's written. But he just took his own time and never did open his mouth to me. Never did say a word but give me that ticket. When he give me that ticket I wanted to tell him he better come on cause he's gonna have to give me another. Cause I was late on a call. And when I got there the baby was born and the baby was dead. And I showed it to the judge and he turned and told that policeman that he think he done a wrong deed holdin me there. "Did she tell you that she was on her way to a call?" He said, "Yes, she did." "And you still helt her there and didn't say anything about it?" "Well I was just givin her a ticket." He said, "Well let me ask you this," the judge says to him. "How much was she speedin?" "She was in a thirty-mile zone makin about thirty-one or thirty-two miles an hour." And made me lost about fo'ty minutes right there. In a thirty-mile zone. White policeman. About that time I don't think they had any blacks. That must've been somewhere in 1959.

I don't know how the baby died but really the baby hadn't just died. See what I mean? But the fact is this—I didn't get there. No tellin what might've happened. But that did happen.

rents didn't say anything about it. They was really upset the baby naturally but they knew they had to get me from the church. She didn't have a hard time in labor so they said. The labor was real easy I would say. But the fact is I wasn't there. And I told him within three minutes he could've said, "Well you go on," and gotten my tag number and given me if he was gonna give me a ticket, and give me one later. Cause that was an emergency. I showed him my permit and my bag cause when I'm lookin for patients like that I carry my bag in the car. Cause I keep my permit in my bag. I showed him my permit and my bag. The judge called him down but that policeman never apologized. You know that policeman wasn't gonna do that. That was too like white.

I remember once—must've been about fo o'clock in the morning—I delivered twins out in Mobile Terrace. One weighed three pounds. The other weighed three and a half. I know to put em in the hospital. I got mother up right quick and got my babies with some hot water bottles. Flat whiskey bottles with warm water in it and put it around em and cover em up real good. I called the hospital. It was the General Hospital then or was it the City? The City Hospital went to the General Hospital and from there on to South Alabama. These were black babies. I had called em and told em I was bringin these babies in.

Well when I got to the desk with em I told em about it. She went in to let em know I was there. So finally she came back waitin on somebody else to come. And then comes the doctor. Now they stood there and here me standin with them lil babies and they stood there lovin and huggin. They paid me and the

babies no attention and there I'm standin with those li}
So finally I said, "Is nobody gonna wait on these babies: _
said, "Well why didn't you say somethin about it?" I said, "You
didn't ask me." I said, "You're askin me why didn't I say. Why
didn't you ask me what did I have to say?" I had been standin.
You know those lil babies if you don't put em in the incubator
they'll die like that. I'm standin up there and didn't want
anything to happen to em. Been up all night and that was gettin
to be around seven-thirty or eight o'clock in the mornin.
They're standin up there laughin and carryin on. Certainly they
were white. Then they realized what I had. I was standin there
right over that box with them babies. The nurse didn't do a
thing. And I had done called em and told em I was bringin em
in. Then I stood there. I bet you I stood there near an hour with
them lil twins. So finally they came and got em and put em in
the incubator. That was not too long after I started workin.

They were prejudice. They didn't pay us too much
attention. They didn't care anything about no big black
womens and no lil bitty black babies. If you were black period
they didn't care too much about you. I told that nurse and that
doctor that I believe you all majored in the wrong thing. Now I
have always spoke up where speakin up needed to be. It wasn't
ugly. It didn't mean to be biggity or uppity. I told em that they
work so slow I was afraid for the lil infants. "I was just watchin
you all over there and I think you majored in the wrong job."
They walked up and they come back and said for somebody to
get them babies. It took somethin like that to kinda lift em up. I
was a lil girl, almost looked like a lil bitty girl cause I started
doin midwife work young. Looked like a lil kid.

There was one time I had complications after a delivery. It was, she had a hemorrhage. She had a hemorrhage. And she hemorrhagin too much and I knew it was too much. And I said, "We're just gonna take her on out to the hospital." So we did call the ambulance and carried her right on to the hospital. This patient had been to my house twice because she thought she was in labor and fixin to have the baby. When she found out that she wasn't, not knowin that she wasn't supposed to, she says to herself, "I'm gonna take me a couple a Bufferin so I can sleep. I get so tired from these contractions." You know there are certain times that you have contractions two or three days befo you deliver. All right, when she went in labor—I don't know how many she had taken durin the time between times she'd taken em, and I didn't know she'd taken em until.

So when she came on over to have the baby, time come for her to have the baby, she came on over to my house and she had the baby, oh—about an hour and a half after she got there. No trouble whatsoever but that aspirins had her blood so thin she had a hemorrhage and it wouldn't clot. It's got to clot. So I picked her up and carried her on to the hospital. The doctor told me if any complications where to bring her with the paper he gave her when she was havin her prenatal care. That is what I have to have. So I carried her on down there and when I got her down there they had to do whatever they did to clot the blood to stop the flow.

The doctor who had given her her prenatal care was outa town but there always is three doctors in the office together. The one that was on call that night was not there, couldn't be found. They couldn't get in touch with him. By the time we found him, when they did got in touch with him, we had done carried her to the hospital and the doctor that was on duty there at the hospital done the work. The child had gone to sleep and everything was beautiful.

So when he finally got there from his party or wherever he had been, the other doctor told him what happened. "She was delivered by a midwife and had a hemorrhage and had to be brought in." I was still there in the waitin room. I was sittin over here waitin and no light. One lil light was sittin there and it must've been around two-thirty. So he come in. He came in and told mostly the wall how mad he was. Cause he was openin the do' and turnin around shuttin the do' when he said how mad he was. But it was referred to me. "I'm so goddamned mad I don't know what to do." I had never seen him befo. Didn't know him. Now he was comin in the do' to tell me off. He came on in and drug his chair up and he had a seat. Drunk. Got him a chair. Drug it up right in front of me. And he said what he wanted to say.

Then I said what I wanted to say. And then I said again what I wanted to say. "You listen at me. We're gonna listen at each other." "I'll have you arrested—brought that dead woman in here." I said, "What dead woman? Who is this?" says I to him. I said, "Who am I talkin to?" says I to him. This is Dr. So-and-So Jones. I don't know what his name is. "This is Dr. Jones." I said, "Well, Dr. Jones, I didn't bring you a dead woman in here and if she done died I want to know that." He kep talkin. All at the same time he just kep talkin. He got on his knees and I just sit there. He said everything that come up. He give it to me and I give it to him. I didn't raise my voice but if he give it to me I give it to him.

I said, "Go back there and ask the doctor and the nurse what happened." He just got afraid for that. "No, she ain't dead but she was about dead when you brought her in here." I said, "I was talkin to her all the way. She wouldn't talk if she was dead." "You don't know what you're doin nohow." I said, "Well, doctor, let me tell you. I've always been taught that if any complications occur for me to take em to the doctor and if you're the doctor on duty I brought her to you just like I was taught to do. I did my duty and when somethin else come up I had to bring her to you. That's what I done and I got her here on time." He said, "I'm gonna have you—I'm gonna have yo license taken. You know I can." I said, "All right. Suit yo'self." That's exactly the way I talk cause he was askin for it. "And futhermo, I done called the police." I said, "I'll be sittin right here when they come. I'll be sittin right here," says I to him. "I'll be sittin right here." And he'd start out the do'—to show you he was drunk—he'd start out the do' and afterwards he'll think of somethin else he'll come back and say somethin else. He'll start out and he'll come back. "I'm gonna have em come in here." "They is go'n arrest me for what? Doin what I'm supposed to do?"

Finally he saw he wasn't gonna get ahead of me on that. He got down on his knees right in my face, holdin his head like that. "You uncompetent nigra woman. You don't know what you're doin. If you want to deliver any mo babies go back to Africa where you come from. Go back to Africa where you come from." He got on his knees right in my face. Right in front of my face. I stood up then. I said, "Let me tell you one thing, Dr. So-and-So." I said, "Let me tell you one thing." I couldn't sit down and tell him. I had to stand up. I stood up and I says, "You done gotten me riled up now. I don't belongs in no Africa no mo than you do. I was born and raised right here in America. If you want anybody to go to Africa to deliver babies, *you* go. I belong here." That's exactly what I told him. I wouldn't have told him that but he pulled it outa me. I wouldn't have. I knows I wouldn't. What come up come out. I said, "Wait a minute befo I let you talk, you're gonna hear my story. I'm not comin from or goin back to no Africa. If you want anybody to deliver babies in Africa, *you* go." I sho did told him that. And I was through with it.

When I got home I got to thinkin about it and I got bigger and bigger and bigger. I really didn't get furious until I got home. It sunk in. To keep from breakin down stompin in my house cryin, I thought about Mrs. Davidson over in the Boa'd a Health. It was beginnin to be about eight o'clock and that's when the Boa'd a Health opens. So I called the Boa'd a Health and got the supervisor and told her about it. She said, "What was wrong with Dr. Jones?" I said, "Dr. Jones was drunk. Probably had been partyin all night." I said, "That's exactly what was wrong with him cause he was on his knees in front a my face and I had to turn my face to keep from smellin his breath. I didn't want to smell it. I hate whiskey breath." When I told her what he said—"If you want to deliver any mo babies go back to Africa where you come from"—she said, "Onnie, he didn't say that. Don't you tell me that. He didn't say that." I said, "Yes ma'am, Mrs. Davidson, that's exactly what he said."

She said, "Put that phone down and get on out to this office." And she hung up.

I got dressed and I got down there and she made a tape of exactly what was said, what was done, how it was done, everything. It's right there in the Boa'd a Health. Made a tape. And she consult him about it. I stood up on my own two feets and I told Mrs. Davidson. He had no idea I was gonna go to the the Boa'd a Health with that. Nothin ever come of it. I know Mrs. Davidson carried it further than she told me. I know Mrs. Davidson did. She carried it much further than she told me.

But they say he's a good doctor. Downright good doctor. The onliest thing that cooled me off, they tell me he come in his office, would have a drink like that and get on his white nurses. That's the way he do his white nurses the same way. He jumps all over em. That's just him. He's just that type of man. And then that cooled me off inside. Really did. I've seen him several times since then. I don't look for an apology. Mrs. Davidson and all thought he was gonna do that, but I got to just say— that's doin too good to give a Negro an apology like that. White man like that don't apologize to Negroes. They're not good enough in themselves to do somethin that good. That's the only trouble I had. I wish I had a chance to talk to him about it and laugh about it. It's been fo years ago. It's been fo years ago cause that baby's fo years old. The mother's fine.

It got up to the point about ten years ago that I was doin so many white girls the doctors didn't like it. After I started doin a whole lot a white girls, the doctors think the midwives are takin the work away. As long as I was doin a lot a po black girls they didn't care, they didn't say anything about it. But when I started doing a whole lot a white girls, nice outstandin white girls, then that's when they started complainin. Said I was takin their money. In fact that's what they said. My patients have come and told me what the doctors said. Said we didn't know what we was doin. We was black. We was ignorant. Because we're black we're ignorant. And we didn't know what we're doin. "Why would you want to fool with them when we got all this equipment here in the hospital? Why would you want to stay home?" If we was havin trouble I could see that's what they would think but we are not havin no trouble. Midwives are not havin any trouble deliverin that baby with home delivery. Doctors just use that as a perch. We're not messin up on jobs and doin a lot a things we don't know what we're doin. It's not that.

Doctors had to go to school for so many years and did all that hard work and then midwives come on who didn't have to put all that hard work and deliver about as many babies. Now that has been spoken right here. In Mobile. From a doctor. He told one or two of my patients that when they was tryin to get their papers filled out that they can have a baby at home.

One a my patients told me that the doctor said if she was financially po he would send the slip to her, but if she could pay for it, he was not gonna send a slip for her for home delivery. If you are financially po I'll give you the slip that you needs for a delivery at home but if you've got the money, no. That has been said over and over. They tried that a lot a times when nothin was wrong. If they tell her now "I don't like you stayin at home cause yo somethin's wrong, blood pressure way back up, you got whatcha call this, that, and the other"—that's one thing. I understood that very well. And I'm sho they did too.

Now this Dr. Johnson has never said anything but somethin good. He was a white doctor. I went there two or three different times with white patients when they started takin their prenatal care. I went once because the doctor said, "I'd like to meet her. I'd like to see what she's like." I would send all a my patients to him because he gave no trouble about the home delivery. All right he died. Then I had to start huntin another doctor because all the other doctors at that time wouldn't give em away. There were just some that would and some that wouldn't. But it wasn't like they all had froze on me.

So Dr. McMillan was glad to receive my patients. Glad to see their condition and if they're eligible for home delivery. He was glad to do that. But the other two doctors got behind him cause I sent him so many. "We two could be doin that work ourselves." It was three doctors in that office and Dr. McMillan is the one who did my white patients. So they got behind Dr. McMillan and written to the Boa'd a Health on account of his insurance and the association said he wouldn't be able to do that anymo. When it happened like it did, he even told me that he was sorry. But he is a member of that insurance group and whatever the group says he has to go along with. It wasn't his fault. I think he told it like you have a meetin and you bring in what's happenin, what you heard about the situation of medicine and all such as that. They picked up on what Dr. McMillan was doin and they sit down and discuss it and put a stop to it. So that broke that up. They had rotated around among the white guys not to do it and they all bein a member of the same insurance, they have to do what one say do or the chairman say do. The white doctors passed it in their convention and in their rules—they stopped every one of em from giving the slips for home delivery. Stopped every one of em. Sho did.

When my white doctors stopped givin me slips for my white patients, I had to end up usin black doctors. I had no alternative to do then but to contact my black guy and that was Dr. Blake. I asked Dr. Blake and he told me to come over and sit and talk to him. Him and I talked just like you and I and I explained it to him and he sit there and listen to the whole story. I sit and talked to him and told him what I was up against and he just looked at me and says—the first thing he said to me after he sit so long and listen at my story—he said, "Onnie, God must've sent you to me." I said, "Thank you, nothin else but God." And he said, "I'll be glad to." I said, "I'm so glad I'd like to cry." I said, "When I get home I'm gonna sit down and call my patients and tell em what I got. And I probably will be callin you to give you names at the office."

So I went back and I started callin my white girls, my seven white girls that I had on list and I told em about it and I told em who he was. I said, "Now he's a black man." They said, "What's the difference? Ain't he a doctor?" Said, "He's a doctor with his license, ain't he?" That's what they told me. The other doctors just mens too. And a man ain't but a man and a doctor ain't but a doctor be he black or white. Man or woman. Just so they know what they're doin to give me my prenatal care so I can stay home and have my baby." I had two or three prejudice husbands that wouldn't let their wife go to the black doctor. I lost two or three of that kind by bein prejudice of the black male.

They started goin to him just like that for their prenatal care so they could stay home and have their baby. I prayed over it many days. I thought it was gonna cause some race trouble. But it worked out fine. My girls said they didn't want nobody, white, blue, or black, to be no nicer. Don't want to go to nobody no nicer. They told that everywhere. They told goin and comin how nice he was. Couldn't be no better. No white doctor couldn't give em no better attention. So in about three weeks from there Dr. Blake called me and said, "Onnie, I got good news for you." I said, "What is that, Dr. Blake?" He says, "There's a female doctor will be in town next month. A black, female doctor here and I know she'll be glad to work with you and yo patients." So they're the only two now that's here for my white girls, their prenatal care.

There hasn't been but one midwife for the last fo or five years and that's me. It's been just me for fo or five years. They outlawed midwifery some time ago. I couldn't tell you exactly why they did that but they told me all over Alabama there was not—not only in Mobile County, and Mobile, Alabama—but they said they wasn't gonna license any mo midwives. They didn't tell me why. They was not gonna license anymo midwives after the ones they already had faded out, retired, or died. This was the first year that they didn't give me a permit. They was goin to retire me after this year. No warnin befo. That's what made me so furious about it. The nurses that worked in the field behind me, you know for my babies, they the time. They said, "Onnie, I don't think they're plannin on givin you yo permit for April." I said, "Well, honey, if that bein the case they hadn't said anything to me about it." They hadn't gotten to me, around to me with it. I don't know about it. I waited for takin it to em. I was tryin to wait to see what they were gonna say to me about it. Never did until I called in to repo't a new patient. My last permit was expired. It said expired in June.

So when I called down there to repo't in a baby, must've been in June. Three mo babies I had to turn in cause they had engaged me to birth em. Mrs. Pete answered the phone and I told her I just wanted to repo't some patients that I had. She said, "Onnie, are you still takin patients?" I said, "Why not, Mrs. Pete? Nobody I told me I couldn't." All at the same time I was thinkin what I had heard. So she said, "Well wait a minute. Let me talk to Mrs. Camp." Mrs. Camp said, "Onnie, you didn't know it?" I said, "Well how was I to know it when you didn't tell me?" she said, "Onnie, you hadn't got a letter from Dr. Manley?" He's the overall chairman of the Boa'd a Health situation. "No, ma'am, Mrs. Camp, I hadn't got a letter from Dr. Manley. In fact I hadn't heard from you in a long time about anything." "They didn't tell you last year when you taken yo physical exam?" "No, ma'am, nobody told me about that." "Well I tell you I talked to Dr. Manley. I have to see why Dr. Manley hadn't sent you a letter cause, Onnie, all the midwives in Alabama aren't gonna get permits this year." I said, "Well all right. That's quite all right with me if that's the way they want to do it but I hate to be left like some Indian that didn't know anything about it as well as I've done through the Boa'd a Health."

All a my good work that I've done. Didn't I deserve better than that? That long I've been working for the Boa'd a Health and didn't have any trouble. I think bein under the supervision of the Boa'd a Health I did a fair honest job with em. I did what I was supposed to have done. No trouble or anything. Finally about three weeks or a month later I got the letter from Dr. Manley. Just letting me know that they had a boa'd meeting some time ago and the boa'd meetin consisted of they would not give permits to any mo midwives. I was throwed out.

Mrs. Davidson told me—my old supervisor—she says— must've been in 'eighty or 'eighty-one—"Tell you what I want you to do. I want you to write a letter to Dr. Manley, a nice letter in your own way and tell him how you feel about yo'self as a midwife and what you would like to do as a midwife." I took her at her word. I written Dr. Manley a real nice letter. I told him, "I know you know how old I am, Dr. Manley, but I don't feel my age. I don't work compared to my age. I just couldn't tell you what I feel like as a person or what age. I would be mo than glad if you would not take my permit from me at least until I was seventy-five if I continue to feel like I'm feelin now."

That was fo years ago. I'd say 'eighty or 'eighty-one she told me to write him that letter. Mrs. Davidson did. And I write him that letter and I know that he was gonna let me carry it till that seventy-fifth year if I lived that long. He wasn't gonna interfere with it. Cause the law said after these midwives that's already licensed retires or dies we wasn't gonna license anymo. Well I ain't dead yet and I hadn't retired. And I'm gonna work until I'm dead. I could do plenty mo work. I wish I could live a hundred years and deliver babies.

If they hadn't've taken my license this year I would have loved to carry two mo years if my health would allow. But if it starts failin or I start getting weak from age they wouldn't have to pull me off. I'd come off. I don't think they did me justice by not givin me my license as long as I feel as well as I am, although I'm an old lady. They're not gonna stop me from doin the gift that God give me to do. The Lord hadn't quite give me the answer but all I'm sayin is that God don't aim for me with the experience He give me and the talent He gave me, He don't aim for me to let man, white nor black, kill it unless my health failed on me. He certainly has used these hands a lot and as long as my health and strength will allow me, I aim for these hands to be used again. I don't want no man stoppin these hands from doin what says the Lord. I don't need a permit to deliver no babies. If God tell me not to do it I won't do it.

I know they cain't stop a daddy from deliverin his own baby. I wouldn't be a bit surprised if I was asked to he'p a daddy. I'm not gonna sit back and not do it. I don't care who know, I go down to he'p em. They cain't stop me from goin there. I don't be goin there on no license. I be goin there as a friend to he'p that husband deliver his baby. That's a way I can legally get around. I'm gonna do that as long as I can. The Lord Himself got to come and tell me not to. Cause I don't go there to take in charge like I was when I was licensed. I sit there and look at that father and tell him what to do and what not to do. I can still get around it. They didn't say I was not supposed to deliver anymo. They said they wasn't gonna issue me a permit for 'eighty-four and my permit expired about three months ago. I'm not their responsibility, you see what I mean. I've delivered only one baby since my permit expired and they don't know that. I just had two patients call to engage me. Three. One yesterday and one today—white—call to engage me for em. One yesterday and one today. So you see how my work grows.

I have gotten to the point in my life now, that I can look back and see that there has been a change. It has changed so much until you can really enjoy it now. Lookin back and seein where we done come from. And I waits because God ain't gonna let you go wrong. If you depend on His leadin and His guidance He's not gonna let you go wrong. You've got to have patience and wait on God and He will lead you through yo problems, yo misunderstandin's, and yo way where you think it's so dark, right around the co'ner is light. I know that and I lives on that. I have seen so many changes. There has been so many changes and I know there are still changes to come as long as there is the world. There are changes to come, better all the time, just gradually comin. All you've got to do is have patience and wait.

I tells even my patients that. Usually a lot a times when they get in labor they wanna have that baby right now. They want to get rid of it right now but all I could do is sit down and quote Scripture to em and tell em that you cain't hurry that baby. He's comin. "I'm tired a this. I'm tired a this baby. I want to get rid a this here." Just be patient and wait. The time will come much better. You'll have a better, easier time and everything will turn out so much better than you have in yo mind, you wanna dump it right now. I tell em that all the time. So many of em, two-thirds of em I do reach in that stage. Every once in a while one that I cain't reach.

I never will fo'get, I had a black girl once and she was in labor and I had delivered about three or fo chil'rens for her. One day she was just carryin on with her contractions. She didn't want to hurt. She was just carryin on somethin ridiculous. I said sit patient and wait and pray. "I done prayed. You told me that last time I had a baby to pray." I said, "Didn't you get through all right? Didn't God lead you through it?" I said, "Well you just as well to have patience and wait with this one because the way you're talkin and the way you're soundin, in the sight a God, He's gonna show you that you gonna wait. And you will have a much easier, shorter time if you get in yo mind, it's my baby and God's gonna let me have him in due time. When the minute and the hour come, yo baby will come. Until then you just makin yo'self uncomfortable tryin to do what you cain't do until the time comes."

I would say to black people that are bitter to take yo time. You cain't hurry God. That was my point. There's a song that we sing, You cain't hurry God. Wait on Him. Be patient and wait and that's what I got—patience and I wait. A midwife like me, they just take their time and let God work the plan.

I let God work the plan on my life and I am satisfied at what has happened to me in my life. The sun wasn't shinin every time and the moon wasn't either. I was in the snow and the rain at night by my lonely self. Plenty of times it wasn't cold but there was rain enough that I had to drive outside of the road and wait for it to slack up so I could see my way. The night Hurricane Camille went through I got a call from Eight Mile, Alabama, which is twenty-two miles or mo out. The wind then was a hundred and seventy-five miles an hour and I got out in that storm and went to Eight Mile to deliver that baby in back of a fruit stand. It was rough but you know what? I taken it with a smile and I enjoyed it. When I was really deliverin babies in all my times, lateness of the hour and the earlies of the mornin didn't bother me. I just went when I was called. There has been a many dreary nights but I didn't looke at em as dreary nights. I had my mind on where I was goin and what I was goin for.

Whatever I've done, I've done as well as I could and beyond. If I had went on I believe I wouldn't've been no mo successful bein a registered nurse or a doctor. I've had several people to tell me that you should've been, you should've been a doctor. I cain't say I wished I had done that because I'd be neglectin the blessin that God give me if I say that. I believe God pulled out all of his blessin's on me and I appreciate em and put em to good work. So I'm satisfied at what I've done. I'm satisfied at what has happened in my life. The only thing I wished I had've had was mo general education. But not anyway that I would've been a real rich doctor or a great big high nurse. Although I didn't get that I'm satisfied. Perfectly satisfied at what my life has done for me. I was a good midwife. One of the best as they say. This book was the last thing I had planned to do until God said well done. I consider myself—in fact if I leave tomorrow—I've lived my life and I've lived it well.

Afterword

In July 1995 the eighty-five year-old woman who called herself my "black mother" passed away. She and I had collaborated on a book about her forty years as a "granny" midwife in Mobile, Alabama. In 1989 this book was published as *Motherwit: An Alabama Midwife's Story*. But much more than a book came out of our collaboration. During the course of our project and its publication, a most extraordinary relationship developed between us—women from different races, different generations, and entirely different cultural backgrounds. Her death caught me off guard and brought me up short, because she had indeed become a mother to me. Despite her age, I never thought of her as an old person who might be near death. She was one of the strongest forces in my life and a heroine in my eyes. How could she die?

I met Onnie Lee Logan in the summer of 1984, through the family she was working for as a maid. My cousin had recently married into that family and had encountered Onnie on visits to his in-laws in Mobile. Onnie had talked for years about wanting to write a book about her experiences as a midwife, but she needed help. My cousin thought of me. I was the aspiring writer in the family, and I had already planned to travel to Mobile the summer following my college graduation, so it was no trouble to meet with her.

When we met one hot summer day in Mobile, I was taken aback. She was by no means the imposing figure of a midwife I had imagined but was instead a tiny, seemingly frail woman with birdlike eyes that darted everywhere and took in everything. I was not prepared for the booming voice that greeted me or the powerful personality that left me awestruck.

At the beginning of our relationship, we made for an odd couple: an elderly black woman employed as a domestic for more than half a century, and a twenty-one year old white girl, a Harvard graduate and a native of the affluent Birmingham suburb known as Mountain Brook. I knew within moments of meeting her that she had the stuff of which books are made; she declared that I was the one to help her.

"You is the one," she told me. "I been praying about this for fifteen years. I was gonna write this book if I had to scratch it out myself, but the Lord done fixed it so I don't have to. I can give my story to you. You'll know what to do with it. You is the one."

Rarely in my life have I felt so chosen or so lucky. Here was a woman who had never finished high school or fully learned how to read and write, yet she had determined to create a book about her life's work. "I want to show that I knew what I knew—I want somebody to realize what I am," she said.

She was also determined not "to die with it." At age seventy-three ("more or less"), she was afraid of dying with her experiences untold. "I don't want to go under ground and have all that covered up," she said. "I don't want it buried with me. I want to leave it behind in black and white."

This undertaking was no less urgent a mission than the many she had been on to bring new life into the world. And in this case, I was to be her midwife. Contributing to this urgency was the letter she had received from the Mobile County Board of Health in March 1984, three months before we met. It abruptly informed Onnie that her permit to practice as a "granny midwife" would not be renewed that year.

Alabama began licensing midwives in 1919, when it was clear that the state's poor, black, and rural population made the midwife a necessity in the absence of any alternative. ("It was the midwife or nothin.") In a black community like the one Onnie grew up in, your granny, or "grannymother," was the woman who had delivered you and first put her hands on you. Later, "granny" became part of the official term for lay midwives who had no medical training. When Onnie applied for her midwife license in 1947, she had to take a course from the Board of Health that instructed her in such basics as how to make the mother's bed sanitary and how to sterilize scissors on a wood-burning stove.

In 1976 Alabama prohibited the licensing of any new granny midwives, but allowed those already licensed to continue practicing at the discretion of the individual county boards of health. Onnie had been the last granny midwife in Mobile County for the previous four years when her license was revoked. Explaining that there was no longer a "need" for granny midwives in the state of Alabama, the letter thanked her for her thirty-eight years of faithful service and wished her the best of health in the coming years.

"Nothing in my life has ever made me feel so little," she told me. "When my husband came home, he had to pick me up off the floor. Fact is, I'm still trying to get up. It set me back that far."

The desire to do a book was part of this effort to pick herself up off the floor, to explain the meaning and significance of who she was and what she had done.

Throughout that summer, Onnie and I spent about two hours every day taping her stories. Her narrative poured out in a torrent, with little prompting. All she needed was someone to receive her story. The more I worked with her, the more this began to seem like a sacred trust.

By the time *Motherwit* came out in August 1989, *Life* magazine had published an excerpt, and the *Today* show had filmed a feature spot. But the most important adventure we had was a cocktail party celebrating the book's publication. Sponsored by the Haunted Bookshop, a local institution that many years ago hosted the first book-signing party for Harper Lee's *To Kill a Mockingbird*, this event set the stage for a small-town drama that revealed a great deal about the complicated dynamics of race and class in Mobile.

It all started when I asked the three white women for whom Onnie had worked as a maid if they would supply the food for the party. I put my request first to Mrs. Simpson (as I'll call her), because she was Onnie's primary employer at that time, and it was through her family that I had come to know Onnie. A transplant from the North and a prominent patron of the arts, Mrs. Simpson was well known for embracing civic duties and complaining about Southern lethargy. I thought she would welcome the role I offered her.

I was wrong. Mrs. Simpson told me that I was taking this party way too seriously; that she didn't expect many people to come or stay very long; that some cheese straws and brownies from a local bakery should be sufficient. When I told her that I *wanted* to take the party seriously and that it was up to us to make this a special event in honor of Onnie, she told me I needed to be realistic.

I did not turn to "Mrs. Mears," Onnie's most long-term employer, because she was by then an elderly woman—the same age as Onnie, in fact. But there was a "Mrs. Williamson," for whom Onnie often worked part-time. She gladly agreed to take charge of the food, and she enlisted the help of Mrs. Mears as well.

Then I got a strange call from Mrs. Simpson. She had not meant that she didn't want to help with the party. And as Onnie's main employer, she thought she should be the one in charge. We could leave everything to her.

I accepted her belated offer and never told Onnie about Mrs. Simpson's initial attitude. All she knew was that her employers were bringing the food, and this was all I ever wanted her to know. On the Friday afternoon of the party, these three white ladies arrived early with their silver trays and serving pieces. They spent the evening passing hors d'oeuvres and replenishing crackers while Onnie stood at the front of the bookshop greeting her guests, many of whom were black. It was a complete, if momentary, reversal of traditional Southern roles.

At one point the owner of the store stumbled into one of these white women, wandering among the bookshelves at the rear of the building. She looked stricken. When he asked her what had happened, she told him, "Oh, nothing happened. It's just that I've never in my life seen black people and white people together at a cocktail party."

I do believe it was a historic moment for the city of Mobile, when some of the more prominent members of the white community found themselves at the same party with some of the more prominent members of the black community. And Onnie Lee Logan had made it happen. Her conviction that her life story was worth telling had turned the world upside down.

But this historic moment did not come without repercussions. On Monday morning when Onnie arrived at the Simpsons', another maid was already there. This was Mrs. Simpson's way of telling Onnie, who had worked for her for the last twenty years, that she was fired. A certain section of *Motherwit* in which Onnie describes Mrs. Simpson had apparently done the damage. By now the book was circulating, and many people in the affluent suburb of Springhill, where all of Onnie's white employers lived, were laughing at what Onnie had said about Mrs. Simpson. I imagine that Mrs. Simpson felt publicly humiliated and personally betrayed, especially after her active contribution to the cocktail party.

The passage in the book that referred to Mrs. Simpson was so brief that I had all but forgotten it by the time the book was published. It evolved after I had asked Onnie what it was like to work for white Southerners. I was thinking specifically of Dr.

and Mrs. Mears, who lived in one of the showplaces of Springhill, a white-columned mansion perched high on a sloping front lawn, with extensive gardens and a little house out back where Onnie had lived.

But the answer I got to my question was surprising.

"I never had as much trouble outa the Southerners....Hadn't never had Mrs. Mears to talk to me or treat me like I have been treated by somebody that's not a Southerner...." Well, everybody knew who that "somebody" was.

With her open contempt for Mobile's Southern ways and Southern residents, Mrs. Simpson had thoroughly alienated herself from the community. ("She thinks these Southerners is trash....Cain't get em to do nothin but sit down.") Yet this lady from the North, despite her supposed superiority and enlightenment, had not treated Onnie well or been supportive of the midwife career that gave so much meaning to Onnie's life.

I had thought this was too important to leave out, especially because Onnie's Southern employers had treated her so well. The Mears had encouraged her midwife work and allowed her to leave the job—even during big dinner parties— whenever she got called by a woman in labor. When she did get a call, Onnie would leave the Springhill mansion to go deliver a baby in a two-room shotgun house in a poor black neighborhood. As a physician himself, Dr. Mears took a professional interest in Onnie's work, and they often discussed it. Onnie had nothing but kind words to say about the Mears and her forty years of service to them.

Had I foreseen the impact of that paragraph about Mrs. Simpson, I would never have asked for her help in the first place. Even so, it was hard to feel guilty about her hurt feelings. As far as I could tell, only when she saw an opportunity for her own self-aggrandizement—when she learned of Mrs. Williamson's and Mrs. Mears's involvement—did she agree to help with the party. And then, of course, she wanted the spotlight. Her behavior only confirmed what Onnie had said about her.

But Onnie was uncomfortable about incurring the wrath of the white lady and felt that she had upset the normal balance of her life. When she called me over to read the offending passage to her, she acknowledged having said the words but reproached me for including them. After all, she had asked me not to put anything about the Simpsons in the book. I argued that she was not to blame for simply telling the truth, and I was not to blame for doing my job as an editor—Mrs. Simpson was to blame for being who she was. Onnie dismissed this argument with a wave of her hand. Then I tried to tell her that she didn't need to be anybody's maid anymore, but she rejected this idea as well. Besides, what most rankled her was the way they had fired her after more than twenty years of being not just their maid but a part of the family. Onnie particularly remembered the week of Dr. Simpson's malpractice trial, when he had wanted her to come every day and sit in the front row of the courtroom. Finally, I told her that for a black woman like herself, writing a book had been a momentous and extraordinary act of self-expression. She couldn't expect that it wouldn't change her life.

Apart from the rift with Mrs. Simpson, however, the book really did not change her life. She didn't let it, as I learned during the filming of an Alabama Public Television documentary on Onnie's life. The cameras and crew were set up on her front porch, and we were in the middle of shooting when Onnie's husband, Joe, pulled into the driveway in his pickup truck. Forgetting completely about the cameras and crew, Onnie got up from her chair and went bustling into the house, saying she had to see after Joe. I followed her inside to ask what was wrong. Nothing was wrong; she just had to fix Joe his lunch. In amazement I followed her back to the kitchen.

"You're not going to fix Joe's lunch *now*, are you?" I asked.

"Of course I am, honey. I always fix Joe his lunch at this time of day."

"But today? When the television people are here? Can't Joe go get himself some lunch somewhere? Couldn't he go to Popeyes to get some fried chicken? Just this once?"

She stopped. "Let me tell you one thing," she said. "Joe can't eat no Popeyes fried chicken. That would tear his stomach up from now till the end of this week." (Joe did have a problem with stomach ulcers.) "But now let me ask you this," she said, confronting me as she always did when I was being "young and stupid," as she often called me. "Why would I stop doing what I have always done? This is how Joe and I get along. I ain't about to stop being who I have always been. Not at this age."

It was perhaps the most important of the many lessons she taught me. It was the same thing she had tried to tell me when I told her that she didn't need to be a maid anymore. In all of her wisdom, Onnie knew better than to change the way she conducted her daily life, or the terms of her marriage and relationships with other people, just because a little celebrity had come her way. In a society in which so many people abandon themselves completely at the merest hint of fame, Onnie held fast to herself. Extraordinary events exploded around her like fireworks, but when the sound and light show was over, she remained intact. Her life continued as before: she played a prominent role in her church, she tended her husband and family, and once every week or so, she polished silver for Mrs. Williamson and arranged flowers for Mrs. Mears. Onnie had too good a grip on herself to abandon that self or be anything other than what she was.

"I'm just a little black girl that God has blessed," she explained to me once. "That's how come I'll never get the big head. I can't take credit for the blessings He give me."

She always said the same thing about her midwife work: "I'm just using the hands that God lent me for a short while to use in His name."

This humility existed side by side with a very strong sense of self-worth. I will never forget telling her about the *Norton Book of Women's Lives*, an anthology of excerpts from the memoirs of such important women as Simone de Beauvoir and Anne Frank. Onnie Lee Logan was among them.

"This means you'll go down in history," I told her.

"Honey, I am history," she said.

I tried to express the strength of Onnie's character when I spoke at her funeral. It was on a Saturday at the Truevine Baptist Church on Dr. Martin Luther King Jr. Avenue, where I had been once before with a film crew from the *Today* show, who were trying to capture Onnie's religious faith on tape. The program for the funeral, the Homegoing Celebration for Sister Onnie Lee Logan, called for three "expressions" from a neighbor, a friend, and a member of the church. I was the friend.

The service lasted three hours and was punctuated by four rousing numbers from the gospel choir, the Truevine Cathedral Ensemble. During the first number, "I called on the Lord," Onnie's sister—her only surviving sibling—became highly agitated, stomping her feet, shaking her head, and waving her arms. One of the nurse's aides, in a starched white uniform and cap, came over from a nearby pew and began ministrations. She fanned vigorously, loosened a collar, offered Kleenex, and hovered in attendance until the singing was over. She came back several times throughout the service to render her assistance.

When it was my turn to speak, I wanted most to convey how this woman, who started off as my collaborator, had ultimately become my "black mother." I told of the time I had been in a car wreck and broken my kneecap. "I'm coming on out to you, baby," Onnie had said as soon as I called her. She stayed with me the whole day. She had to accompany me on each trip to the bathroom, because I could not sit down without someone to lift and hold the cast on my leg from hip to ankle. She gave me a sponge bath. She dressed me. She fixed my lunch. She helped me in and out of bed and sat by my side to keep me company. Then she came back the next day to do it all again until my father came from Birmingham to get me.

Helping others defined the essence of Onnie Lee Logan. From the time she was a little girl in Sweet Water, Alabama, playing in the yard with her homemade dolls, Onnie had had visions of helping people. Because in Onnie's imagination, her particular doll was always sick. And she had asked God to let her be a person to help others.

She also asked to tag along on her mother's visits to the sick and to women in labor. Not allowed in the room, Onnie would peek through the cracks in the houses and watch her mother deliver the baby and cut and tie the cord. "And I prayed to God to let me do those kinda things." But her forty years as a midwife were only part of her lifelong mission to serve others in any way she could.

There was the time that Onnie and I happened to be in Birmingham when my grandmother, who was dying of lung cancer, was rushed to the hospital and put in intensive care. She was in the final gruesome stage of the disease, when the cancer was literally eating her alive. The doctor had said she would probably not last through the night, and might go within the hour.

"I don't know if I can face it," I told Onnie.

"Oh, yes we can," she said.

When I knew Onnie was going with me, I knew I could endure the ordeal. Former patients of hers had said the same thing about labor and childbirth. Once Onnie arrived, they knew they could do it. She could handle birth, death, and everything in between with a skill, grace, and intelligence that truly did seem to come from that "higher power" she was always talking about.

We three went together to my grandmother's room—my mother, Onnie, and me. When we got there, my grandmother reached out her hand from what I knew would be her deathbed. She reached not to my mother, her daughter, or to me, her granddaughter, but to Onnie, a black woman whom she barely knew, as if some supernatural radar were guiding her toward the strongest person in the room. A mere wraith of her former self, she clutched Onnie's hand as if for dear life. My mother grabbed Onnie's other hand as we gathered around the bed. Three generations of white women were deriving their strength and courage from the lone black woman, who kept up a continuous conversation while my mother and I tried to conceal our devastation.

My gaze fixed on the two hands lying on top of the covers—one black and gnarled due to lifelong labor and delivering more than one thousand babies, the other white and fragile, not only from cancer but from years of inactivity, with painted red fingernails from a recent trip to the beauty parlor. Onnie Lee Logan and my grandmother were both Southern women nearly eighty years old. But my grandmother was the only child of well-to-do parents who lived in an exclusive neighborhood. She had led a privileged life as a daughter and then as a wife. Onnie Lee Logan was the fourteenth of sixteen children who grew up on a farm in the Alabama Black Belt during the Depression. Her life of hard manual labor began when she was a child, picking cotton in her father's fields. Her hands had done everything. They had milked cows and picked cotton; they had delivered babies and "laid out" corpses for burial. My grandmother's hands had done little. I mainly remembered them as holding the cigarettes she had started smoking when she was fifteen, the day she was initiated into her high school sorority. As I stood there and watched Onnie coaching my grandmother through death as she had coached so many other women through childbirth, I knew I was witnessing the tragedy of one kind of womanhood and the triumph of another.

When my grandmother died, it was to me the final succumbing of a frail life that had been defeated long ago. But when Onnie died, I was shattered. The Onnie I knew was invincible. She had possessed an almost superhuman ability to deal with anything life presented her and to overcome any obstacle. The hardships of being a black woman in Alabama had not stopped her; they made her stronger. ("All that Depression wasn't paid too much attention to. We just managed and went through it.") Despite everything that stood in her way, she achieved a success known to few: she did what she wanted to do with her life. At the end she could say, "The world doesn't owe me nothin. I have fulfilled my life. If I had a second chance, I would do it all over again exactly the same way," she said. "I loved it that well." With her lifetime of perseverance and her ultimate triumph, she was to me the life force itself. "Young and stupid," I had not thought death would lay her low; nothing else ever had.

In many ways, she was the one person in my life I could turn to as a pillar of strength. She was also my role model for a strong woman, a model that my own white Southern culture had failed to provide. When I lived in Mobile, I often called Onnie in distress. "Come on over to me, baby," she would say. When I got to her house she would be waiting at the front door to take me into her arms. "Poor little white girl," she would say. "You got so much education stacked up to here, but you don't know nothin, do you?"

One of the sagest pieces of advice she ever gave me was: "Stay normal." I can hear her now, saying, "Don't start acting crazy like a lot of young peoples do, trying to make themselves happy, running around, drinking too much, taking up with whoever. Stay normal. You hear me? Keep yourself ready for when that right thing come along."

There are the things I tried to say at her funeral. Perhaps my most special memory, which I did not share, is when the book came out and I took that first copy over to Onnie's house.

"Read some of it to me, baby," she said, and I did.

"That's in the book?" she asked when I finished.

I nodded.

"That's nothing but my own words," she said. "That's exactly what I said to you."

"I know it, Onnie. I thought I told you that's how I was going to do the book."

"The whole book's like that?"

"The whole book."

"You mean you didn't write it? It's all my own words?"

"It's all your own words."

She looked up at the ceiling. "Thank you, Jesus," she said. Then she looked back at me. "God bless you, baby."

In the last hour of the funeral the minister offered a "message of comfort," which was really a sermon based on the text of Onnie Lee Logan's Christ-like life. Then came the "reviewing of the remains" and the recessional, when all of her family members stood up to file out of the church. Until that moment, I had never realized what a large extended family she had. I was particularly struck by the group of young black males, ages eight to seventeen, who passed by. These must have been her grandchildren and great-grandchildren, the ones who called her "Ma Dear." I had never met them but had heard her hollering at them sometimes when I called her house. She would chew them out good, tell them where they could find something to eat in her kitchen, and then resume her conversation with me. Now tears were streaming down their faces. They all clutched white washcloths that they were not too proud to use.

Beside me Amanda Williamson, another of Onnie's many poor little white girls, was also sobbing. When the time came for Onnie's sister to stand up, she let out a primal wail of grief.

"Oh, Onnie, what is life going to be like without you?" she sobbed. This was everyone's question.

My one consolation is that Onnie did not "die with it." Telling her story was the final thing she wanted to accomplish before she died, and she did it. I was simply the lucky one to receive the gift from her soul. I am the one forever transformed by coming so close to the power and beauty of an extraordinary woman.

—Katherine Clark

This Afterword was originally published in the September/October 1999 issue of the *Oxford-American* under the title "Reflections on the Last Alabama Midwife."

CPSIA information can be obtained
at www.ICGtesting.com
Printed in the USA
LVHW090141210921
698328LV00001B/3

9 781611 879261